Healing
Skin Disorders

Healing Skin Disorders

Natural Treatments for Dermatological Conditions

Acne ◆ Eczema

Psoriasis ◆ Shingles

and More

Andrew Gaeddert

North Atlantic Books
Berkeley, California

Published by

North Atlantic Books   Get Well Foundation
P.O. Box 12327   8001A Capwell Drive
Berkeley, California 94712   Oakland, California 94621

Cover and book design by Catherine E. Campaigne

Printed in the United States of America

Healing Skin Disorders: Natural Treatments for Dermatological Conditions is sponsored by the Society for the Study of Native Arts and Sciences, a nonprofit educational corporation whose goals are to develop an educational and crosscultural perspective linking various scientific, social, and artistic fields; to nurture a holistic view of arts, sciences, humanities, and healing; and to publish and distribute literature on the relationship of mind, body, and nature.

Healing Skin Disorders: Natural Treatments for Dermatological Conditions is also sponsored by the Get Well Foundation, a nonprofit organization whose purpose is to educate the public and health care providers about natural therapies that are complements to Western medicine. Get Well Foundation operates a clinic, publishes books, and sponsors seminars.

Library of Congress Cataloging-in-Publication Data
Gaeddert, Andrew.
    Healing skin disorders : natural treatments for dermatological conditions / by Andrew Gaeddert.
        p.   cm.
    Includes bibliographical references.
    ISBN 1-55643-452-9 (pbk.)
    1. Skin—Diseases—Alternative treatment—Popular works.   2. Skin—Care and hygiene.   3. Naturopathy—Popular works.   I. Title.
RL85.G34 2003
616.5'06—dc21

                                                        2003010377

*This book is dedicated to Carol Gaeddert
and all the wonderful people
at Health Concerns*

Contents

Introduction

Healing *Skin Disorders* focuses on herbal, nutritional, and lifestyle approaches to treating skin disorders. Many of these are drawn from Chinese medicine. The encouraging news is that if these factors can be addressed, it is possible to overcome your skin condition, even if conventional Western therapies have not been effective.

There are many causes of skin disorders. Some conditions are genetic; others are caused by emotional upset. The most common negative emotions—anxiety, worry, sadness, fear, and anger—can cause skin conditions by leading to interruption in circulation, which can impede waste elimination. Let's say you are very angry, then your face might become red. Over time, unless you can let go of the anger, your blood vessels may constrict, causing tension and lack of blood flow. This holding on might lead to constipation, which would lead to toxins being released through the skin, producing acne or other eruptions.

Thus, we strongly recommend both daily exercise and stress reduction as a part of our program.

Poor diet is another factor in skin conditions. If you are upset, you may not have the time or the energy to eat healthy foods, or your whole life might be on the go. Foods contributing to skin diseases include greasy or fatty foods, excessive sweets, including cookies, pastries, cakes, pies, and other desserts, fruit juices (due to their excessively sweet nature), dairy products, wheat, alcohol, caffeinated beverages, food additives, and prescription and recreational drugs. Therefore we urge you to strive for a clean diet.

Some people are constitutionally sensitive, resulting in allergic skin conditions. If your skin is exposed to excessive wind (which is drying), coldness, heat, dryness, or damp weather, you may develop skin disorders. You may also develop a skin condition due to infections or animal bites, especially insect bites, which may cause dermatological disorders. Finally, chemicals in the workplace or home can be the problem.

In *Healing Skin Disorders,* you will find lifestyle and other suggestions as well as herb and nutritional supplements that can be self-administered or that require a professional's guidance. Whenever possible, we advise consulting a health professional trained in herbs and nutrition. When it comes to your own health, even the most highly trained practitioners seek the help of others. Why? Because it is very difficult to be objective about one's own health. A professional may be able to reach a diagnosis differently from that of your medical doctor. They may have different explanations for why you have a skin condition and how you might heal. For example, an herbalist trained in TCM (Traditional Chinese Medicine) might take into account not only the appearance of your skin, but your appearance as a whole. They might ask questions that you haven't thought of before, such as about your perspiration, your stools and urine, your appetite, occupation, or sensations of warmth and cold. They might look at your tongue or take your pulse or touch your skin. Of course, for a thorough biomedical diagnosis it's also important to see a dermatologist, whenever you notice skin changes.

Herbal medicine has been used for thousands of years. The reason for using herbs rather than drugs is that herbs work more gently, and therefore cause fewer side effects. Recently there have been many misleading articles in the press about using "standardized" herbs. These are expensive herbal products promoted for a single constituent. This misleads the public into believing that there is a single active ingredient in an herb or an herbal blend. Most serious herbalists reject this claim because they know that an herb may contain dozens, and sometimes hundreds, of active components. The recent controversy about St. John's wort is an example. German scientists once assumed that hypericin was the only important ingredient, and therefore they did all they could to isolate this single component. Later, scientists speculated that a different constituent called hyperiform was responsible for St. John's wort's antidepressant effects. However, having a guaranteed amount of one of these constituents does not guarantee a better or stronger product, therefore, most trained herbalists prefer to use whole St. John's wort or will at least suggest adding the whole herb to a "standardized" product. As we will see later in the text, St. John's wort offers far more than antidepressant effects, and in fact, its primary use in the West for hundreds of years has been for counter nerve pain such as that in shingles and sciatica. The important fact is that herbs are not drugs, which is why they may provide healing through complex actions.

In terms of Chinese medicine, skin conditions are thought to be caused by imbalances of the lung and liver, although other organs can cause them as well. Although Chinese medicine is very complex and difficult to understand, the following chart is meant to describe what personal habits and qualities, and what symptoms Chinese medicine associates with your skin condition.

Hot & Dry Conditions

- Itching with heat sensation
- Symptoms worse with hot weather
- Bright red papules or macules
- Smoking
- Being easily angered
- Constipation (can also be due to cold)
- Being easily upset
- Being prone to afternoon slump
- Dark urine
- Being loud and dominating
- Yellow phlegm
- Fast pulse rate
- Early and heavy menstruation, bright red blood
- Burning and dryness of the skin
- Itching
- Thirst
- Tongue, red and dry
- Pulse, rapid and may be floating

Dampness

- Swelling or edema
- Blisters
- Food allergies
- Being worse in moldy damp environments
- Intestinal gas, bloating, indigestion
- Being heavy, overweight
- Pulse, sluggish
- Sadness or depression (feeling weighted down)
- Worry
- Dull sensations
- Food intolerance
- Hay fever
- Tongue, pale with thick coating
- Pulse, slippery quality

Cold

- Sensations of coldness—condition worsens in winter
- Dry skin (blood deficiency)
- Itching worse in cold
- History of anemia
- Chronic loose stools
- Tongue, pale
- Pulse, slow and sinking

Note to Practitioners

One of the nice things about treating skin conditions is you can see the progress right in front of your eyes. My observation is that patients tend to be more patient when seeking help for their skin in comparison with how quickly they expect relief from other disorders. Many of the clients we have successfully treated have been unable to be helped by other CAM (complementary and alternative medicine) providers. I attribute this to several things. One, my approach takes into account three important factors: lifestyle, nutrition, and herbs. We often pay attention to how compliance can be best achieved. For example, in the American clinic, patients usually do best when given herbs in pill form, as long-term treatment may be required for satisfactory results. Frequently we recommend herbs internally and topically. I hope that *Healing Skin Disorders* will give practitioners more confidence and help their treatments to become more comprehensive for the good of their patients.

Chapter 1

Tips for Healthy Skin

The health of your skin is directly related to your overall health. In this chapter we discuss ways to improve your skin and general health. These suggestions are utilized in our clinic and in many other clinics across the country. Herbs and other natural therapies work more slowly than conventional drugs; therefore, it's important to give the approaches mentioned in this book ample time to work. A good rule of thumb is one month of treatment for every year of illness. Thus, if you've had a skin condition for over ten years, it may take one year of faithful use of herbs and supplements for you to experience a major improvement. In our clinic, we often see patients with difficult skin problems who have not been treated successfully with Western medicine. If they consistently follow all our suggestions, they are usually able to see some results in one to two months. A major improvement or total resolution is often possible in six to twelve months.

Food and Water: Foundation for Healthy Skin

The skin is the largest organ of the body. Like the rest of the body, in order for the skin to be healthy, proper nutrition is necessary. This means that intake of both water and food needs to be adequate in amount and nutritionally sound.

Drink Enough Water

Water transports nutrients, helps eliminate toxins, and modulates body temperature. The superficial layer of the skin, the epidermis, is able to hold a great deal of water, thus making it elastic enough to help maintain the body's fluid and electrolyte balance. If you're continually dehydrated, your skin is depleted of its water content and starts to show signs of dryness and cracking. I suggest drinking at least sixty-four ounces of water per day, either hot, lukewarm, or at room temperature. You may drink filtered water or mineral water. Either buy water flavored, or use a wedge of lemon or lime or cucumber to make it more flavorful. Chinese medicine and many European traditions hold that cold beverages and food injure the digestive system and so these should be avoided. Reducing or staying away from caffeinated beverages such as coffee and soda, in addition to alcohol is also a good idea, since caffeine and alcohol are diuretics and can increase the body's need for water. For coffee, substitute green tea. Caffeine-free herbal teas (as described at the end of Chapter Two) can be used instead of water.

Eat Wisely

The age-old recommendation of following a diet that emphasizes fresh fruits and vegetables, lean meat, fish, and poultry is particularly important for persons with skin problems. According to Chinese medicine, there are a number of skin conditions such as eczema and acne that can be caused by an improper diet. This means the diet that you have is not suitable for your constitution. In Chinese medicine, a food is characterized by its energetic property. If you tend to have a hot condition, that is, feel persistently hot and have red rashes that worsen during the warmer months or in warmer climates, you should eat foods that are cooling in property. These include watermelon, grapes, cucumber, pears, mung beans, and soy products (if you're not sensitive). Additionally, reduce or eliminate your coffee intake because coffee is warming. Instead, drink water or beverages that are cooling, such as peppermint or chamomile tea.

If you have itchy skin and are tired and pale, you may require more foods that "build blood." Eating meat, especially liver, is the best way to build blood. Nettles (an herb) is recommended by Western herbalists to build blood. Cook the fresh leaves the way you'd cook spinach, or put one to three tablespoons of dry nettles powder in soup or stew, or make a tea with one teaspoon of powder in eight ounces of water, simmer for five minutes, then steep for ten to fifteen minutes. Nettles are available in health food stores. Chinese herbalists suggest the herb *tang kuei,* red dates, and longan fruit to build blood. If you have skin boils, poor digestion, and/or joint pain, pearl barley porridge can be used to improve the skin and digestion. It may also be helpful to increase your intake of fatty fish, which contain oils that have anti-inflammatory properties, and are thus considered beneficial for a wide range of skin conditions and constitutions. Eggs are a good source of vitamins and protein. Cook them before eating since raw eggs

Sensitivity	Substitute
Milk and other dairy products	Lactaid milk, goat milk, rice milk, nut milk
Coffee and other caffeinated drinks	Green tea, herbal tea, coffee substitute
Sugar, fructose, fruit juice	Honey, whole fruit, real maple syrup, rice syrup
Eggs (chicken)	Eggs from turkey, duck, ostrich, turtle; egg substitute (made from potato)
Corn	Blue corn, alternate grains
Wheat	Rice, buckwheat, other grains
Soy	Miso or tempeh may be tolerable
Tomato, pepper, eggplant, potato	Other vegetables
Chocolate	Carob
Alcoholic beverages	Alcohol-free wine and beer, herbal relaxants (see Chapter Three)
Fermented foods	Herbs and spices as seasonings
Meat and fish	Organic meat that does not contain antibiotics or hormones Fresh water fish
Aluminum cookware	Ceramic, glass

Reprinted from *Healing Digestive Disorders* by Andrew Gaeddert.

prevent the absorption of biotin, a vitamin necessary for healthy skin. Also, eating eggs raw places you at risk for salmonella poisoning.

An essential part of the diet that is frequently overlooked is oils. Healthy oils include fish, olive, flax, avocado, walnut, and black currant. These oils contain anti-inflammatory components and thus are important for controlling the allergic and inflammatory responses that occur in conditions such as eczema, psoriasis, lupus, rheumatoid arthritis, and asthma. While supplementing with healthy oil it is important to reduce or eliminate unhealthy oils such as margarine and shortening. These are associated with immune suppression, obesity, increased harmful cholesterol, and other health hazards. Unhealthy hydrogenated oil, oil that's undergone processing, is found in most processed food such as cookies, muffins, bread, crackers, cereal, chips, mayonnaise, and salad dressing. For better health, cook with olive oil, which has not undergone chemical processing, and contains oleic acid, a component that is currently being studied for its usefulness in preventing tumor growth. Instead of commercial salad dressing, use one to two tablespoons of olive, flax, or walnut oil. Eat fish such as salmon, mackerel, sardine, tuna, and eel, which are high in ecosapentanoic acid (EPA) and decosahexaenoic acid (DHA). These omega-3 polyunsaturated fatty acids have, among other health benefits, anti-inflammatory effects. If you have an active skin disorder such as psoriasis, eczema, lupus, dry skin, brittle nails, hair loss, you might also consider using fish oil supplements if you are unable to eat fish a few times a week. Choose a product that contains both EPA and DHA, such as cod liver oil. (Do not use cod liver oil if you are pregnant or planning to become pregnant, due to the high vitamin A content.) Therapeutic dosage is at least 3 to 10 grams a day. To illustrate the importance of adequate dosage, one of our clients, Justine, had lifelong psoriasis. A nutritionist put her on a vitamin and fish oil program, which helped her symptoms somewhat. When she saw us for an herbal consultation, we found that she was not taking enough of the fish oil. We recommended an herbal regimen, and six capsules per day of fish oil concentrate, as well as eating fish a few times a week. Within a few weeks Justine's skin condition improved dramatically.

Vegetarians who have skin disorders should also try to incorporate fish into their diet, or use fish oil capsules. Oils that contain gamma linoleic acid (GLA) such as primrose, black currant, and borage oils can also be used. Of the GLA oils, I prefer black currant oil, as it is not as warming as evening primrose oil, and is also used as food; for example, jam is made from black currants. Daily dosage is 3 g (follow label instructions carefully). The better products contain a small amount of vitamin E to prevent rancidity.

Many foods and families of food are known to trigger skin reactions. These reactions range from classic allergy symptoms whereby the immune system responds to an individual sensitivity. The table below lists foods that cause reactions; note their substitutions. If you're unable to identify your trigger food(s) either on your own or through a food journal (see below), you can try going on an elimination diet. This involves eating only lean meat and vegetables, preferably organically grown and naturally raised, for two weeks. Then add foods one at a time to see if they cause symptoms.

If you're having difficulty assessing and modifying your diet, it may be useful to keep a food journal. For two weeks, everything you eat is logged. Keeping a food journal creates awareness for what you're eating. In addition record any skin changes. You may be surprised by the amount of junk food you're indulging in, especially between meals. A food journal can also help identify which foods are causing or contributing to your skin problem. Culprits include alcohol, sweets, shellfish, fried foods, and spicy foods, particularly those seasoned with chili peppers. Dairy products (such as milk and cheese), foods that contain gluten, especially wheat, as well as yeast-containing foods, such as bread and pastries, are also known to cause skin problems.

If you're unable to identify trigger foods, try eating a diet of lean protein, vegetables, and rice and millet for two weeks to see how your skin responds. Gloria, one of our clients, experienced remarkable improvement in both her psoriasis and her digestive system with herbs and this diet. Denise, an eczema patient, successfully identified wheat as the food that was exacerbating her symptoms. She was on this diet for two weeks, and when she added wheat, her rash quickly worsened. She made a choice to not eat wheat after realizing the effect on her skin.

Improve Your Digestion

Many of our clients who have skin conditions also have poor digestion. This isn't surprising since greasy skin, boils, and inflammation are signs that elimination is not normal, because toxins are being excreted from the skin, not through the urine and bowel movements. In Chinese medicine, the skin is connected through the energy channels to the large intestine by way of the lungs. Persons who have skin problems often started out with chronic digestive difficulties, with constipation and loose stools as the two most common symptoms.

Constipation is usually due to not getting enough fluids. Drink more water, especially hot water, since according to Chinese medicine, hot water promotes peristalsis. It's important to note that "fluids" not only refers to liquids, but also to foods that are high in water content, or that moisten the intestines. These include fresh vegetables and fruits; dried fruits such as prunes, figs, and raisins are also helpful. Flaxseed, at one to three tablespoons daily, freshly ground, or flax oil on salads and vegetables can be used as well. He shou wu, also known as foti, is a Chinese herb that nourishes the hair and has a moistening effect on the bowels. To make a tea, boil one tablespoon of the herb for ten minutes and let it steep for five to ten minutes. Cindy complained of dry skin and constipation. In addition to recommending an herbal tea containing *he shou wu,* we suggested that she take flaxseed with oatmeal and fruit every morning, and supplement with fish oil. Within three weeks she was much more regular. Over time, her skin required much less moisturizing. If you want to try it, take the tea daily for several months; however, if you have loose stools, do not use this herb. If you have heat signs (see Introduction), you might consider using dandelion tea. Simmer two to three teaspoons of the root in eight ounces of water for ten to fifteen minutes.

Chronic loose stools or diarrhea can be due to a variety of reasons according to Chinese medicine. A cold constitution (signs include constant cold hands and feet) or low energy (qi) are among the more common causes. One very helpful remedy is colostrum, which is mother's first milk after giving birth. Follow instructions on the label, and if this doesn't work, you can usually safely double the dosage of most colostrum products. Also recommended are traditional Chinese herbal formulas such as Six Gentlemen and Source Qi, which help boost the energy, and warm the system. Other remedies include Digestive Harmony, a formula I developed that can be used for occasional loose stools, cramping, gas, and abdominal bloating. For more information, consult a health professional, or refer to my book, *Healing Digestive Disorders.*

Clear Your Liver

Our liver converts everything we eat and drink into nutrients for our muscles, hormones, blood, and immune system. The liver stores vitamins, minerals, and sugars, and produces bile, which rids the liver of waste products, and helps break down and absorb fats in the small intestine. The liver, in addition to the kidneys, clears the body of harmful substances. These substances include chemicals, alcohol and drugs, toxins produced by bacteria and fungus, and waste created by the breakdown of protein. If you're overweight, have a history of hepatitis, or have used alcohol, pharmaceutical, or recreational drugs, or have been on steroids, estrogen, or oral contraceptives, or have been exposed to pesticides, cleaning solvents and other chemicals, you have an extra reason to detoxify your liver. Detoxification can be accomplished by eating fresh fruits and vegetables as often as possible, exercising regularly, eliminating or minimizing your use of alcohol, avoiding recreational drugs, and reducing or avoiding exposure to harmful chemicals such as household pesticides. Sweating is also a good way to detoxify your system. This can be done in a bath. (See "Try Healing Baths" section, later on in this chapter.) Specific herbal and nutritional products to aid the liver are mentioned in Chapter Two: Skin Herbs and Nutrients.

Nourish Your Immune System

Healthy skin reflects an adequately nourished immune system. If your immune system is not working well, you are susceptible to increased infections, including those affecting the skin. Microbes such as bacteria, viruses, funguses, and parasites can take advantage of a deficient immune system and cause disease. You can nourish your immune system by eating a healthy diet that includes plenty of fruits and vegetables, along with sufficient protein. Drinking green tea instead of coffee is also helpful, since green tea contains antioxidants, which protect the body from "free radicals," atoms or groups of atoms that impair the immune system. Taking antioxidant supplements such as carotenoids, vitamins C and E, in addition to selenium and zinc benefits the immune system as well. Other ways to nourish the immune system are exercising, having a daily stress reduction program, quitting smoking, and reducing or eliminating alcohol.

Stephen had a chronic bacterial infection of the skin, which was controlled with Astra 8, an herbal formula that boosts the immune system. When he stopped taking the formula the infection recurred, requiring him to take antibiotics. We suggested a comprehensive program of exercise, stress reduction, and herbs applied topically, in addition to maintaining the Astra 8. Over the next year, Stephen was able to reduce his antibiotic use by seventy percent.

Check Your Thyroid

The thyroid gland is an important organ of the endocrine system. It secretes hormones that are important for controlling body metabolism. Poor thyroid function can lead to disease, including skin conditions. According to Brota Barnes, M.D., author of *Hypothyroidism, the Unsuspected Illness,* poor thyroid function can contribute to the following skin conditions: boils, impetigo, cellulitis, erysipelas (a strep infection of the skin), acne, itching during the winter months, eczema, ichthyosis (scaling), lupus, and psoriasis.[1] Dr. Barnes recommends measuring your basal metabolic temperature as a simple way to check your thyroid function. This is done by inserting a thermometer under your armpit for ten minutes before getting out of bed in the morning over three or four consecutive days. An average temperature below 97.8°F may reflect low thyroid function, known medically as hypothyroidism. Temperatures above 98.2°F may indicate hyper-thyroidism, or elevated thyroid function. Do not measure your temperature during a cold or the flu, or if you have other con-ditions that may raise your temperature. Menstruating women should take their temperature during the second, third, and fourth day of their period, since during ovulation basal temperature fluc-tuates. If your basal body temperature is consistently low or high, notify your health professional, who may then want to order tests and recommend thyroid medication or other treatment. If your body temperature is low but your tests are normal, consider the following therapies, especially if you have fatigue, depression, low libido, water retention, dry skin, hair loss, paleness, decreased sweating, or slow wound healing: eat plenty of seaweed, which is rich in iodine; take zinc (15 to 60 mg per day), selenium (200 mcg per day), and iron if you're anemic. Daily exercise can also help, but be careful not to exhaust yourself. Your holistic prac-titioner may be able to suggest specific herbal blends or thyroid glandular extract to address thyroid problems.

Diane had psoriasis and was always tired and cold. She had a history of anemia and low thyroid function. In addition to herbs and fish oil, her holistic physician recommended natural thyroid. Almost immediately after taking it she felt warmer and began to see improvement in her psoriasis, which hadn't been responding to topical steroids.

Quit Smoking

Smokers frequently have worse skin than non-smokers. Ciga-rette smoke contains thousands of chemicals, including formalde-hyde, DDT, and arsenic. These chemicals disrupt the circulatory system and cause the blood vessels that supply oxygen to the skin to contract, thus damaging the elastin of the skin. Carbon monoxide, which builds up in the blood of smokers, robs the body tissues of oxygen, adding to damage of the skin. The many perils of smoking are well known and well documented. If you smoke, and care about your health, not to mention your skin, you would do well to quit. If you are trying to quit smoking, it is a good idea to enroll in a local program for support. Acupuncture can be an useful adjunct to stop-smoking programs.

Participate in a Stress Reduction Program

Many skin conditions are triggered by stress. Flare-ups may occur in anticipation of a stressful event, during the stress, or afterwards. Major stresses include familial changes (such as death of a spouse or change in marital status), work difficulties or changes in employment, retirement, moving, or even holidays. What causes a flare-up in one person may be invigorating for the next. I once read a story about two singers. One continually suffered panic attacks and was afraid to perform, because before a show, her palms would sweat, her heart would race, and she would feel butterflies in her stomach. However, when another singer was asked how she *knew she was ready* to perform, she remarked that her palms would get sweaty, her heart would race, and she would feel butterflies in her stomach.

In this day and age, each of us is subjected to stress on a daily basis. Some persons cope with stress better than others. For those who don't, it is only a matter of time before their health is affected. Participating in a daily stress reduction program is a good way to reduce the negative effects of stress on our body. I try to get my clients to commit an hour each day to a program that combines exercise and stress reduction.

The exercise should be one you enjoy doing by yourself or with a friend. Exercise increases circulation, which helps eliminate waste and promotes healing, thus making your skin look better. Even while exercising, you should protect the skin. Do not use makeup because the pores become blocked when you sweat. If you have long hair, tie it back so that you can sweat freely. To prevent contracting or transmitting skin pathogens, use your own towel to cover the seat and backrest of exercise equipment, wear rubber sandals in the shower and locker room, never share razors, combs, or brushes. Treat cuts and abrasions as soon as possible. Wear breathable shoes and let your shoes dry out following workouts. Shower after exercising to avoid excessive bacteria buildup.

Reducing stress means doing some form of quiet activity that allows the mind and body to relax. Such activities include meditation, yoga, Tai-chi, or prayer. The key to these disciplines is that they should be done with an awareness of the breath. A relaxation exercise that I have found helpful is the meditation on the following page.

Herbs and nutrients that support the adrenal gland, which helps us adapt to stress, include vitamin C (2 grams per day), B vitamins (choose a multiple B-complex), and magnesium (250 to 500 mg daily). Keep in mind that B-complex vitamins can cause agitation in some people, and magnesium in excess can result in loose stools. Herbal relaxants include kava, valerian, and passionflower, which taken in moderation, can be helpful.

Pay Attention to the Seasons

Ancient people and farmers have always lived according to the seasons. We can follow this example to help preserve the health of our skin. During the summer, avoid exercising outdoors in the heat of the day, and wear cotton clothing and other natural

Meditation with Breath

Sit or lie down with your spine straight. Follow the directions below. Twenty minutes once or twice per day should be enough to reduce tension and improve your alertness and energy level. Over time your skin will thank you.

- Place one hand on your abdomen covering your navel.
- Inhale through your nose, being conscious of your abdomen extending; it may be helpful to repeatedly say to yourself "breathe deeply" during inhalation.
- Hold your breath for a comfortable period, then exhale slowly through your mouth, paying attention to your abdomen deflating; again, it may be helpful to say "relax completely" during exhalation.
- An alternative is the "four times four breath." Breathe in for a count of four. Hold your breath for a count of four, then let your breath out for a count of four. Continue breathing in this fashion for twenty minutes. A more advanced version is to breathe in for a count of four, hold for four, breathe out for four, and hold your breath with your lungs empty for a count of four before breathing in.

fibers that breathe. Drink water and herbal teas to prevent dehydration, particularly of the skin. Do not wash with soap too frequently in summer because soap is drying and actually causes more oil to form on the skin. In addition to a once daily use of soap, splash your face with water, sponge bathe with water only in the armpits, groin, and other areas that have sweat glands, unless directed by your health professional.

During the cooler months humidity drops; therefore, the air is drier. Use mild soap, since astringent soaps can be too drying.

Begin moisturizing in the fall and through the winter to prevent dryness. Wear a hat, scarf, and gloves to protect against the elements. Keep room temperature at 68°; temperatures any warmer remove moisture. Drink plenty of warm beverages such as water with squeezed lemon or lime, or herbal teas.

If your skin suffers from dryness buy a humidifier, and if your skin is oily, consider getting a dehumidifier. Portable units can be kept in the bedroom or used on a room-by-room basis.

Determine Your Skin Type

Finding out your skin type can be helpful in resolving your skin problem. Wash your face, and don't apply cosmetics afterward. After one hour, press a tissue against your forehead, chin, nose, and cheeks. Oily residue on the tissue indicates oily skin; if the oil is found only on the forehead, nose, and chin (called the T-zone), and not the cheeks, you have combination skin. If skin particles are found on the tissue, and flakes are visible on the skin, you have dry skin. You may have flaking areas on one part of your body, and oily areas in other parts. It's normal for the chest and back to be oily, and the legs and feet to be dry.

Know Your Soaps

Soap lifts dirt and oil away from the skin so they can be rinsed away easily. Many commercial soaps contain animal or vegetable oil and other harsh ingredients that may make your skin itch, burn, or feel tight after using. Health food stores carry a wide range of hypoallergenic natural soaps that may be easier on your skin. Transparent soaps often contain glycerin and may be helpful for dry or irritated skin. Lanolin, cocoa butter, and cold cream soaps are designed to both remove dirt and moisturize the skin. Antibacterial soaps not only wash away dirt, but also remove bacteria. These soaps are controversial because they help to spread antibiotic resistance, which means that germs become used to antibacterial remedies, and thus even pharmaceutical antibacterial drugs do not work as well as they once did. Deodorant soaps kill bacteria that cause body odor; they are considered harsh and should *not* be used on the face. Herbal soaps, such as oatmeal or aloe vera, are gentle and contain plant moisturizers; calendula soap is especially good for acne. Make sure to use soap after handling raw meat, before handling contact lenses, or if you are around sick people.

Jan had extremely greasy skin with one of the worst cases of acne I'd ever seen. We recommended a comprehensive program that included washing her face twice a day with calendula soap, taking herbal formula Coptis Purge Fire, and modifying her diet. Her skin breakouts stopped within two weeks. When she resumed her old diet, which consisted of greasy foods, sweets, and soda, the acne came back, convincing her of the importance of permanently changing her lifestyle, especially her diet.

Choose Cosmetics Wisely

If your skin is prone to rashes or is easily irritated, it's wise to use hypoallergenic products. Any product can cause a reaction on your skin, therefore it's important to first test it by applying a small amount on your skin and wait twenty-four hours to make sure the product agrees with you. The common symptoms of contact dermatitis are itching, blotchy rashes, blisters, cracking, and bleeding where the product was applied.

To protect against infection, avoid sharing free samples or testers of cosmetics, and brushes or applicators that have been used by other people. Wash your hands and face before applying cosmetics; apply mascara carefully to avoid scratching your cornea. Close or seal cosmetics to avoid airborne pathogens; store them in a cool, dark place, avoiding direct sunlight, because the ingredients can alter when exposed to sunlight. If you add herbs, vitamins, or liquids to your cosmetics, prepare no more than a one-day dosage. This mixture should be stored separately.

Try Healing Baths

Daily baths can reduce stress and can help heal your skin. Essential oils, herbal recipes, or combinations of oils and herbs can be added to the bath. Essential oils are placed into the bath after it has been drawn. Herbs are usually placed in the tub when it's empty. After getting out of the tub, cover up with towels, and lie down for about half an hour. Putting on relaxing music enhances the experience.

To soak the stress away and help you sleep better, use ten drops of lavender and five drops of marjoram. Lemon balm is also a relaxant: Simmer three tablespoons of lemon balm in 64 oz of water for ten to fifteen minutes, steep another five minutes, and pour into an already drawn bath.

Certain essential oils have been found to be effective for various skin conditions. The following can be added to an already drawn bath.

- ◆ For dry skin use four drops each of geranium and rose, and ten drops of sandalwood.
- ◆ For oily skin use four drops each of cypress and juniper, and ten drops of bergamot.
- ◆ For red inflamed or sensitive skin use five drops of chamomile and two drops each of neroli and rose.

◆ For acne use twenty drops of bergamot, five drops of juniper, fifteen drops of tea tree oil, and five drops of cypress.

The drops of essential oil may be placed in two tablespoons of almond or another vegetable oil (such as olive) and shaken before adding to bath. Oils like almond and olive serve as "carriers," since some essential oils are too strong to be applied directly to the skin.

An oatmeal bath is especially beneficial for dry, itchy skin: Put eight ounces of oatmeal in a muslin bag. Boil it as you would to make porridge, then use the bag to sponge your whole body while in the bath. Commercial oatmeal bath products such as Aveeno are also found in health food stores and pharmacies.

For psoriasis, try a smilax (sarsaparilla) bath: Simmer three tablespoons of smilax powder in 64 oz of water for five minutes,

Shaving Care

Shaving can remove skin and can cause razor bumps, which is known medically as pseudofolliculitis barbae. Razor bumps are more common in persons of African descent and in people with curly hair. The bumps are caused by reentry of coiled hair into the skin. Shaving actually sharpens the hair, making it easier for the hair to re-penetrate the skin. Any area that is shaved can be affected, including the beard, armpits, head, and legs. Stopping, or shaving infrequently is the best way to resolve this condition. But if this isn't possible, then avoiding a close shave might prevent re-entry of shaved hairs. Single-blade razors or special razors that prevent close shaves can be used. Also, try shaving in the shower or right after showering, when the hair is completely wet and soft; shaving creams are also helpful for hydrating the hairs. Shave in the direction the hairs grow, and use aftershave, which closes the pores and soothes the skin from the abrasion of shaving. If you get a nick or cut, or are subject to inflammation, use witch hazel or an aftershave with alcohol. Ingrown hairs can be loosened with a commercially available pre-shave abrasive sponge.

23

steep for another ten minutes, and add to an already drawn bath. Lawrence had psoriatic arthritis (a condition with joint inflammation and skin lesions) with lesions all over his body. He exhibited signs of heat, so we advised him to take daily baths with smilax decoction with lavender essential oil added after the bath was drawn. Lawrence also took internal herbs and nutritional supplements. He stayed on the program for eight months over which he experienced gradual healing of the lesions, and he was able to reduce his pain medication.

To remove flakes and scales, mix half a pound of Epsom salts and with one-fourth cup of sunflower or olive oil and massage your entire body starting with the toes and working up to the face; follow this with a warm bath. (This is a scrub and may take getting used to.)

A detox bath helps draw out toxins from the body: Fill the tub with hot water. Add one-half to one pound of Epsom salts and soak for about fifteen minutes. If you become lightheaded, get out of the tub. Then lie down in the bed and cover yourself with a sheet or towel. This bath promotes sweating.

All herbal teas and essential oils should be used with caution during pregnancy.

Skin Massage or Essential Oil Massage

Whether you massage yourself or have a partner massage you, results will include relaxation as well as benefits to your skin. When massaging you will need carrier oil—an oil in which to dilute the essential oil—since some essential oils can irritate the skin if applied directly. Almond oil is suitable for all skin types; olive and sunflower are good alternatives. Safflower is used when an injury or pain is present. If you have dry skin, combine nine parts almond oil to one part avocado oil. If you have oily skin, consider using hazelnut oil as the carrier. For the face and hair use jojoba oil. For aging skin, consider adding one part wheat germ oil to nine parts almond oil, or use peach or apricot kernel oil. Essential oils can be added.

Protect Yourself from the Sun

The incidence of skin cancer is on the rise; about one million cases are diagnosed each year in the U.S. It should be remembered that sun damage is cumulative, and continued overexposure ages the skin, causing lines, wrinkles, leathery skin, and uneven coloration. Of vital concern is skin cancer. What can you do? Try to avoid the sun between 10 A.M. and 3 P.M. when the rays of the sun are most direct. Whenever possible wear a hat, sunglasses, and clothing that covers your arms and legs. Use a sunscreen with a SPF (sun protective factor) of at least 15. Look for a product that contains ingredients such as PABA (aminobenzoic acid), vitamin E, and aloe vera. PABA has been found to be very effective in preventing sunburn. Sunscreen should protect against both UVA and UVB radiation. Apply at least half an hour before you go into the sun, as it takes time for sun protective ingredients to be absorbed. Don't forget your face, ears, hands, and lips.

Nutrients may offer additional protection from sun damage. One example is green tea. Preliminary studies with hairless mice indicate that green tea may reduce the incidence of ultraviolet-induced skin tumors. This is one of the many reasons for drinking tea instead of coffee. The active ingredients in green tea—catechin polyphenols—have antioxidant and other properties that protect against cancer. Another example is vitamin C. Sheldon Pinnell, M.D., professor of dermatology at Duke University Medical Center, has found that vitamin C, applied to the skin before UV exposure, prevents UV-induced skin damage.[2] This new form of vitamin C, ascorbic palmitate, is fat soluble, and therefore has a longer action than other forms of vitamin C. Carotenoids, pigments found in fruits and vegetables, protect plants from UV rays. They can protect humans in much the same way; thus, it makes sense to eat colorful fruits and vegetables and consider taking supplements containing mixed carotenoids (30 to 50 mg daily). Pycnogenol, or grape seed extract, and other capillary strengthening flavonoids such as blueberry and bilberry support the circulatory system and may deter the breakdown of collagen, such as occurs with aging or inflammatory collagen diseases.

Beware of Photosensitizers

Certain foods, drugs, and herbs can make your skin more sensitive to sunlight. This is known as a photosensitive reaction. The skin may be more susceptible to sunburn, swelling, or rashes. In extreme cases blistering, damage to the blood vessels, and even cataracts may develop. Foods that may trigger a photosensitive reaction are celery, lime, parsley, and wild parsnips. Even artificial sweeteners have been implicated. Ingredients in deodorants, soaps, lotions, and moisturizers can also cause photosensitivity. Drugs are also known to result in reactions in a small percentage of persons. Such compounds include antihistamines, antibiotics, especially tetracycline, oral contraceptives, nonsteroidal anti-inflammatory drugs (such as ibuprofen used as a pain reliever), sulfa drugs, and tricyclic antidepressants. Natural products such as the essential oils of bergamot, cedar, lavender, rosemary, lime, and lemon, as well as St. John's wort may also induce photosensitivity.

Identifying the offending item(s) is usually by elimination, after which avoiding the sun is the best way to prevent recurrence.

For some persons, sunscreen is helpful. Be sure to discuss any medication you're taking with your health professional to check if it is known to be a photosensitizer.

Protect Yourself at Home and Work

Contact dermatitis is a skin rash caused by a substance that comes in contact with the skin. The rash can be the result of an allergic reaction or of the toxic effect of the substance. Common substances include cleaning fluids, paints, turpentine, and latex (found in gloves and condoms). Other offenders are metals such as nickel, as found in watch straps, necklaces, and bracelets. Topical medications such as the antibiotic neomycin have also been reported to cause reactions. Once the substance has been identified, avoiding it is the best way to prevent future occurrences. If this is not possible, then preventive measures include washing your hands immediately after you encounter a known offending substance, wearing protective clothing, such as gloves or goggles, and a protective body suit at work.

Create a Healthcare Team

Just as with any other medical condition, you should always consult your doctor for a diagnosis of a skin problem. That little bump or blotch can reflect a more serious medical situation. It's also important to remember that medications you take can cause skin problems. You can read about your medication in the *Physician's Desk Reference* (*PDR*) or in the *Nurse's Drug Guide*. Talk with your doctor about possibly reducing or eliminating medications that may be causing your skin symptoms.

If your skin condition is not responding to conventional medicine, or if you'd like to try natural remedies, you may want to first consult with a holistic health professional. For some diseases, herbs, acupuncture, or other alternative modalities can be quite helpful. However, serious diseases such as skin cancer or systemic conditions that have accompanying skin symptoms, are best treated by standard medical care, and using holistic techniques to complement Western medicine.

Stay Informed about Skin Medications

It is important to look up all medications you are taking or considering in the *Physician's Desk Reference (PDR)* or *Nurse's Drug Guide,* available at a public library or bookstore. Find out if any of the medications you are taking can negatively affect the skin. For example, many medications cause itching. Meet with your health professional to find out if there are alternatives that will not be harmful to your skin. Before consenting to surgery or other invasive techniques, make sure to ask your dermatologist about the risks, side effects, and the recovery time that is needed. Below is a brief review of some of the more popular skin medications.

Those Taken Internally

Botox—Botox is botulism toxin A. Botulism toxin B is known as Myobloc. While this treatment may be acceptable for people with severe pain disorders, approach using botox for cosmetic purposes or excessive sweating with extreme caution. This is a deadly toxin linked to contaminated food that has been altered.

Concern has been raised as to whether this might weaken the immune system or cause other complications. Muscle weakness, ptosis (eyelid drooping), bleeding, and pain have been observed. Botox wears off after four to six months, and cosmetic treatments tend to be expensive and not reimbursable with insurance.

Antibiotics are useful for skin infections and are also prescribed for acne. While using antibiotics for acute infection may make sense, the long-term use can cause many side effects and complications.

Methotrexate is used to treat abnormal cell growth and is prescribed for recalcitrant psoriasis, rheumatoid arthritis, and cancer. It is toxic to the liver and can cause suppression of the bone marrow, rashes, fatigue, fever, gastrointestinal, and lung complications. It depletes folic acid so if you are taking this medication, ask your health professional about supplementing with folic acid (400 to 800 mcg per day). Tests should be administered to measure liver and kidney function while you are on methotrexate, due to its toxicity.

Cyclosporine is used as a medication of last resort for severe psoriasis and other autoimmune conditions, and the side effects it produces include blood abnormalities, tremor, convulsions, headache, insomnia, night sweats, skin malignancies, and hallucinations.

Inflixmab (Remicade) is an approved drug for Crohn's Disease and rheumatoid arthritis and is undergoing studies of its use to treat severe psoriasis. It can lead to infections, including tuberculosis.

Hydroxyurea is an oral medication that can increase the effects of UVA and UVB light treatments. It may cause anemia.

Steroids (prednisone, cortisone) may be used internally as well as topically. While they stop inflammation quickly, they can thin skin permanently and cause weight gain, nervousness, and bone loss.

Retinoids are derived from vitamin A. Some popular medications include tretinoin (Retin A, Renova), isotretinoin (Accutane), acitretin (Soriatane), tozarotene (Taxoroac), and adalapene (Differin). Retinoids, often prescribed for acne, can cause peeling, redness, and burning, and make the skin more sensitive to light. Often it takes three months or longer to see a beneficial effect, and they are expensive. Isotretinoin (Accutane) is also available in pill form and treats stubborn acne. Not only is this pill expensive, it can cause severe birth defects if it is taken during pregnancy. It may also cause muscle and joint pain, headaches, dry eyes, decreased night vision, and elevated levels of cholesterol and triglycerides.

Alpha Hydroxy Acids (AHAs) are derived from natural products. For example, malic acid is from apples; citric acid is from citrus; lactic acid is from milk; tartaric acid is from grapes; glycolic acid is from sugar cane; and mandelic acid is from almonds. These are available as creams, lotions, cleansers, peeling agents, and facial masks. AHAs increase fluid in the skin and are used to decrease wrinkling and age spots and are sometimes combined with Renitin A to make the skin appear younger. They are available in both prescription and regular (over-the-counter) strength. Like all moisturizers they are best applied when the skin is moist. Redness and stinging are the most common side effects.

Those Taken Topically

Bath solutions such as oatmeal or chamomile can be used to reduce itching.

Calcipotriene ointment (Dovonex)— This is a prescription medication that relieves itching for psoriasis patients. It is a synthetic form of vitamin D. Common side effects include itching, burning, redness, and swelling.

Anthralin is used to treat thick patches of psoriasis. It is contraindicated if your psoriasis is active and inflamed.

Coal Tar has been used for over one hundred years. Over-the-counter and prescription strengths are available to slow cell proliferation (overproduction) and inflammation. The benefits are usually short lived, and it is messy and tends to stain clothing.

Tazarotene is a prescription retinoid that may be used by itself or combined with UV rays. Women of childbearing age should not use it if there is any chance they are pregnant, as it can harm the fetus.

Salicylic Acid reduces itching and scales associated with psoriasis and eczema.

Topical Steroids (corticosteroids)—Topical steroids have been used in dermatology since the 1950s. There are dozens of topical steroid preparations. They are popular because they initially work well for rashes, they are easy to use, and they are not messy compared with other topical applications. As with any topical preparation, it is possible to have an allergy to one or more of the components in the steroid. The most common side effect is thinning of the skin, so that it looks pink or red since the blood vessels are more visible and dilated. Chronic use of topical steroids may result in a systemic reaction with side effects such as edema, weight gain, increased blood pressure, etc. If using a strong preparation, this may develop after only a few weeks. Another problem with steroids is they tend to lose effectiveness if used too often (tachyphylaxis). If you decide to use topical steroids, it is important to use the correct preparation on the correct part of the body. In other words, on areas of the thick skin it may be necessary to use a stronger steroid than on more sensitive areas. For best absorption apply steroids after the skin is moist or well lubricated. Your dermatologist may suggest wrapping your skin with plastic wrap after applying the steroid to increase the topical absorption.

Antifungals—While topical antifungals are often more effective and less messy than herbal remedies, dermatologists often prescribe antifungal drugs internally. While effective, drugs such as ketoconazole (Nizoral), fluconazole (Diflucan), itraconazole (Sporonox), and terbenifine (Lamisil) are toxic to the liver and expensive. It may make sense to use pharmaceuticals for topical administration and use diet and complementary approaches to treat fungus systemically if the fungal infection is not life threatening.

Doxepin (Sinequan) is a tryclic antidepressant used by dermatologist for its anti–itch, sedative, and antihistamine effects. It is useful for patients who keep picking at their skin, not allowing it to heal. Doxepin, like other tryclic antidepressants such as diazepam (valium), must be used short term, as tryclics are highly addictive. Common side effects include drowsiness, confusion, heart palpitations, skin rash, rise in blood pressure, and urination problems.

Skin Definitions

Crust (scab)—Dried blood, pus, or skin fluids on the surface of the skin.

Erosion—A breakdown of the top surface of the skin (epidermis). Erosions are caused by irritation, infection, and pressure.

Lichenification—Thickening and hardening of the skin from continued irritation.

Macule—A flat, discolored spot less than four-tenths of an inch in diameter. Freckles and many rashes are macules. A *patch* is like a macule only larger.

Nodule—A solid bump up to four-tenths of an inch in diameter, which may be raised.

Papule—A solid bump less than four-tenths of an inch in diameter; a *plaque* is a larger papule.

Pustule—A blister containing pus, which is formed from white blood cells.

Scales—Areas of thickened dead epidermal cells, producing a flaky, dry patch. Psoriasis and seborrhea often present with scales.

Scar—A mark remaining after the destruction of the dermis.

Ulcer—A more severe erosion. It is a breakdown of the epidermis and at least part of the dermis.

Vesicle—A small, fluid-filled spot less than two-tenths of an inch in diameter. A blister is a larger vesicle. Insect bites, shingles, chickenpox, and burns form vesicles and blisters.

Wheal (hive)—A swelling of the skin that produces an elevated, spongy area that suddenly appears and then disappears. Wheals are a common expression of allergic reaction.

Light Treatments

Sunlight—Ultraviolet (UV) light kills T-cells in the skin that lead to overgrowth and scaling. While spending time in the sun will tend to help many skin conditions, it is important not to get burned.

Phototherapy narrow band UVB light can be administered in a doctor's office or the "light box" at home. Typically, healing requires three treatments a week for eight to twelve weeks. PUVA and psoralen (topical medication that makes the skin more sensitive to UVA light) is used for twenty or more treatments. Too much PUVA can age the skin and may contribute to skin cancer.

Climatotherapy

Thermal basins such as the Dead Sea, or spas in Florida or the Caribbean, allow treatments consisting of sun exposure in mineral rich air, with bathing in the water for an hour or more a day. It is reported that the mineral content in air and water in combination with stress reduction contributes to successful treatment. If you cannot travel to these remote areas, it may be possible to take mineral supplements and soak daily in Dead Sea salts or other mineral rich bathing products.

Chapter Two

Skin Herbs and Nutrients

Herbs are simply plants that are used in medicine. The reason that herbs are not more popular in the U.S. is they cannot be patented as drugs, and no drug company wants to spend millions of dollars researching something they cannot patent. Until there is research comparing herbs and drugs, we really don't know which is more effective. In the treatment of skin conditions, there are thousands, possibly millions of patients who have not responded to drug therapies. In my experience, many of those patients can be helped with a change in diet and lifestyle, and appropriately taken herbs. It is very important that you get your skin condition diagnosed. The herbs mentioned in this book have been chosen for their safety. As a general precaution, we also recommend not using herbs during pregnancy.

It is possible, although rare, that you might experience an allergic reaction to herbs. If you have history of many allergies or intolerances, it is important to introduce all changes, including taking herbs and supplements, at a reduced dosage. The herbs and herbal products mentioned in this book should be safe for children; however, it is important to reduce the dosage by at least half. If you are on any medications, it is important to take the herbs and drugs at least two hours apart. Herbs are generally best taken on an empty stomach, that is, between meals. Most herbs and other nutritional supplements are best stored in a cool dry place, typically a kitchen or bathroom cupboard. Unless specifically labeled, they should not be refrigerated unless they are brewed as tea. Generally, brewed tea should be kept in the refrigerator or consumed soon after preparing.

Chinese and Western Herbs

In both the West and in Chinese medicine, treatment with herbs has a long history. There are some differences in how they are used. In the West herbs are usually recommended singly or in small combinations of up to five herbs. In Chinese medicine, typically five to twenty herbs will be employed. For herbalists, the advantage of using multiple ingredients, whether in prescribing an herb tea or designing an herbal formula in tablet or capsule form, is to improve results and minimize undesired effects.

Many Western herbalists try to be experts in picking herbs, processing them like old time pharmacists, and seeing patients. In Chinese tradition, these are typically done by several different people, such as the grower or harvester, the processor, herbal pharmacist, and the herbalist.

It is advisable to take herbal remedies under the guidance of a knowledgeable health professional who can select the most effective remedies for your signs and symptoms. Many people who attempt self-treatment do not take the correct products or the correct dosages. The best way to find a professional with experience using natural therapies is word of mouth. If you write to me, I may be able to locate a practitioner in your area. (See Resource Guide at the end of this book.)

It is important to be patient when treating long-standing skin conditions with herbs. There are a variety of reasons for this. One, natural therapies generally work more slowly and with fewer side effects than drugs. Two, certain drugs, especially steroids, make it more difficult for the body to heal, despite producing impressive results in some cases. Three, many of the dermatological clients we see also have other health problems, the most common being digestive (IBS, constipation) and respiratory complaints (asthma, frequent colds, flu). Good holistic therapy aims at improving your overall constitution, and therefore improving all your symptoms over time. One advantage of herbal medicine is that treatment is general; therefore over time you should notice an improvement in your skin and in your overall health.

Herbs may be taken in tincture, tea, tablet, and powder form. In general, I do not recommend tinctures, as they are an inefficient way of consuming herbs internally; however, they work well for topical applications. Teas, tablets, and powders allow you to take a higher dosage of herbs, and therefore they are best suited for internal administration. As we will see later in the book, teas, powders, and tablets ground to powder are also used for topical administration.

For skin conditions, herbal products are more effectively absorbed on an empty stomach with a large glass of hot or room temperature water, or hot herbal tea when recommended. Herbs may also be taken with meals to aid the digestive process.

While using natural therapies, it is possible, though not likely, that you will have a healing crisis. The most common symptoms are a temporary worsening of your skin condition, or you may experience diarrhea or constipation or discharges. To avoid this I recommend starting herbs and dietary supplements at reduced dosages.

It should be pointed out that these remedies are considered dietary supplements, and are not researched in the way that drugs are. Information about these products has been gathered on the basis of historical usage, which includes a great deal of trial and error. Never discontinue prescription medications without consulting your health professional. Even though herbs may be safe and effective, until more is known, we do not recommend herbs during pregnancy.

Herbal Terms and Directions

Decoction—A decoction is tea made by simmering roots, bark, and stems typically for twenty minutes or longer. For whole herbs use approximately one ounce (30 g) of herbs per sixteen ounces of boiling water; strain before drinking.

Chinese herbs—Take as directed by your herbalist.

Herbs in tea bags—Steep in teapot or a cup with a lid on for five to ten minutes.

Powdered herbs—Simmer for two to three minutes and then cover and steep for ten to fifteen minutes and strain. Use one teaspoon of powder to eight ounces of boiling water.

Infusion (dried, cut, and sifted herbs)—Flowers, leaves, and thin-stemmed herbs are steeped with a lid for ten to fifteen minutes. Use one to three teaspoons of herbs (depending upon weight) per cup of boiling water (i.e., with lighter flowers, use three teaspoons; with dried herbs, use one teaspoon). Strain.

Poultice—A poultice is made by adding a small amount of hot or room temperature water to powdered herbs so they are damp. Apply the water/herb mixture to the skin (one-quarter-inch thick) and cover with breathable surgical tape or gauze. (Your herbalist may suggest adding aloe gel for burns and rejuvenation, honey, a natural antiseptic, healing oils or liniments to the herbs.) To keep the poultice warm, wrap a heated water bottle or heating pad in cloth and apply over the poultice. If the poultice irritates the skin stop using. It's important to change poultice at least once per day.

Fomentation (wash)—A cloth soaked in warm herbal decoction or infusion, strained and applied topically over the skin.

Tinctures are liquid alcohol extracts of herb that can be applied topically to the skin as directed by a health professional or internally as directed.

Salves can be made by simmering three to four teaspoons of herb in oil (typically olive, safflower, or sesame) for one hour. Adding beeswax (four tablespoons per one cup) may thicken it if added to warm herbal oil. Stir while the salve cools and thickens. More beeswax can be added if desired.

Bath—Two to four quarts of decoction and/or fifteen drops of essential oil can be added to an already drawn bath. Or add fresh chopped herbs or dried herbs wrapped in cheesecloth as the bath is filling up.

A **Soak** is made by bathing an affected area in a decoction or infusion. Soaks are particularly useful for bruises, sprains, insect bites, and rashes.

Tablets and **Capsules** are the easiest way to take herbs. Typically herbs must be taken at higher dosages than drugs, so it is very important to take this dosage if you want to get the best results. Some herbalists recommend combining two or more formulas to customize your herbal blend. Herbalists usually recommend herbal combinations. If you are self-treating, you may want to use one herb at a time.

Specific Remedies

Aloe Vera—Aloe was first used by the ancient Egyptians for skin infections. It was listed in the U.S. Pharmacopoeia in 1820. Aloe is found in many dermatological and cosmetic products. It is used topically for acne, burns, irritations, seborrhea, and ulcers. It is also used internally for constipation and other digestive disorders. Various concentrations of aloe are effective for a wide variety of skin bacteria and fungus. Aloe extracts also have anti-inflammatory effects. Aloe stimulates wound healing by stimulating fibroblast and connective tissue formation, and aids in the regeneration of new skin. It is easiest to select pre-made products for topical use.

Calendula (marigold)—Calendula, also known as marigold, is one of the premier skin herbs for inflammation of the skin, including acne, eczema, and psoriasis. It may also be used for wounds, burns, and scars. It also has antifungal properties. The easiest way to take this herb is to buy a bar of calendula soap and wash the skin once or twice per day. It may be also used in an antiseptic lotion with goldenseal and myrrh, applied directly as a tincture or poultice.

Capsicum (red pepper)/Capsaicin—Capsaicin is the component responsible for the pungent effects of red (cayenne) pepper. In addition to relieving pain, capsaicin has been used to treat psoriasis. Studies have demonstrated reduction of scaling, thickness, and itching. If you use capsicum, start with a small area. It is not uncommon to temporarily experience burning after administration. This side effect seems to be reduced with continued application.

Chamomile—Chamomile is best known for its ability to treat nervousness, insomnia, and indigestion. The flowers are used externally, as well as the oil made from the flower, for helping to reduce skin inflammations and to heal wounds. Chamomile essential oil is widely used in Europe in shampoos, lotions, salves, and soaps. The constituents azulene and chamazulene have anti-allergic activity. Another constituent, apigenein, has anti-inflammatory activity. Chamomile may produce an allergic reaction in some people who have ragweed allergies. To make a tea, take 1 to 3 tsp of dried flowers, steeped in a cup of hot water, three times per day. To make a bath, take a quarter pound (100g) of dried flowers, steep in a gallon of hot water for twenty minutes, strain, and pour into the bathtub. Use products topically as directed.

Chaparral was traditionally used by Native Americans to treat colds, bronchitis, snakebites, chicken pox, and arthritis. It has also been used topically for bruises, rashes, eczema, psoriasis, dandruff, wounds, and internally for digestive disorders and cancer, and used as a mouthwash to kill bacteria. Chaparral should be used externally and is not recommended internally without supervision of a knowledgeable herbalist, as it may not be appropriate for people with history of liver disease. Make a tea by simmering 24 oz of water and 1 to 3 tbsp of powdered herb for five minutes; let it steep for fifteen minutes before applying topically as a wash.

Clay has been used medicinally since biblical days. It is traditionally used topically to reduce swelling. It has also been used for acne. It is especially good when combined with other herbs. For example, it is usually made into a paste that is combined with a hot herbal tea and applied as a poultice. Take 1 tsp of clay mixed with water, or for stronger effects, herbal tea, and thinly spread over the affected area (one-eighth inch or 3mm thick) and then cover with a thin gauze. In the case of nerve pain or mumps, add St. John's wort oil to clay.

Colostrom is the very first mother's milk. It is rich in factors designed to kick start the infant's immune system. Colostrom can be taken internally to supplement the immune system, and remove bacteria, virus, and fungus. It can also be applied topically for all sorts of sensitive skin conditions. Simply add a small amount of water to powdered colostrom and apply to the irritated area and cover with gauze. This should be changed twice per day.

Coix (pearl barley)—This herb can be used as a food: add six to eight cups of water to one cup of coix and simmer for two hours. It can also be taken as a medicinal herb. For example, one preparation, Coix Tablets, is a modern formula used for acne and shingles, and it contains coix (*yi yi ren*), salvia (*dan shen*), *chimonanthus* (*la mei hua*), oldenlandia (*bai hua she she cao*), rehmannia (*sheng di*), sophora (*ku shen*), calamus gum (*xue jie*), and red peony (*chis hao*). In terms of Chinese medicine, coix is said to remove dampness.

Comfrey contains allantoin, a biological constituent that promotes the growth of new cells. Allantoin is the active ingredient in several over-the-counter and prescription drug products. Comfrey is topically used for skin inflammations including cuts, wounds, and burns, as well as for eczema and psoriasis. It should only be used internally under the guidance of a health professional, as the prolonged internal use of comfrey may be harmful to the liver. For topical administration, simmer 1 tsp of powdered comfrey in 8 oz of water for five minutes, steep ten to fifteen minutes and apply topically as a wash. Add a small amount of water to make a poultice. Powdered comfrey can also be added to aloe vera lotion. Comfrey is not recommended for pregnant or nursing mothers.

Goldenseal is one of the most popular American herbs. It is used topically to treat eczema, ringworm, and athlete's foot. It is used both topically and internally for canker sores, and wide variety of infections. Goldenseal contains berberine, a powerful natural con-

stituent with anti-bacteria, antifungal, and anti-protozoan properties. It is particularly known for its ability to stop infectious diarrhea. Make sure to buy goldenseal from reputable companies
specializing in herbs, as inferior suppliers have substituted cheaper
herbs for the expensive goldenseal root. Typical dosage is two to
three grams per day in tablet form, or topically as a poultice.

Gotu kola (centella asiatica) is used for many skin conditions,
including varicose veins, cellulite, wound healing, scleroderma,
skin ulcers, lupus, perineal lesions, burns, and keloids. It is not
related to the cola nut, and therefore contains no caffeine. Clinical studies have demonstrated excellent or good results in the
treatment of cellulite. In one study of 65 patients taking gotu
kola for three months, 58 percent showed very good and 10 percent satisfactory results.

Gotu kola extract was used internally in studies of patients
with keloids or hypertrophic scars. The extract reduced inflammation or relieved symptoms in 82 percent of the patients. In
several trials involving scleroderma, gotu kola reduced skin indura-
tion and arthralgia symptoms, and improved finger mobility. In
one study of 13 patients, oral administration of 200 mg of gotu
kola was judged very successful in 3 of 13 cases, successful in 8
of 13, and unsuccessful in 2 of 13.[3] General dosage is 60 to 120
mg of extract a day, or 2 to 4 grams of powdered gotu kola taken
in tablets or capsules.

Grape seed extract contains proathocyanidins, (OPCs) which
are beneficial flavonoids that are also found in pine bark. OPC
products inhibit the destruction of collagen. They have been clinically used for varicose veins, insufficient blood flow, venous insufficiency, and other conditions such as cardiovascular disease,
diabetic retinopathy, and macular degeneration. I recommend
Quercenol, a supplement with grape seed extract and other

antioxidants, or Collagenex, containing collagen type II, which nourishes the skin.

Horse Chestnut—Horse chestnut seeds have been traditionally used for varicose veins, venous congestion and inflammation, phlebitis, and by people who tend to bruise easily. This herb also prevents edema, especially lymph edema, treats hemorrhoids, has pain-relieving effects, and helps to heal leg ulcers. It can be used in lotion for the above conditions and for leg ulcers. It is important *not* to use the raw herb as it needs to be specially processed. Look for a product that contains 40 to 50 mg of aescin per tablet or capsule. Take 3 tablets per day. Topical gels usually contain two percent aescin. Follow label directions.

Kelp and other seaweed—Kelp and other seaweed are detoxifying. For example kelp helps protect the body against radiation and heavy metals. Therefore, if you are undergoing radiation therapy or have been exposed to radiation or other toxins, it makes sense to try to incorporate seaweed into your diet. Generally the properties of seaweeds are cooling; therefore, they should be used cautiously with cold signs (see Introduction) or digestive weakness. Seaweed may also be used topically in the form of soaps.

Lavender—Lavender flowers with their beautiful blue violet colors have been traditionally used to soothe the nervous system and to treat skin conditions, such as eczema or psoriasis, that are worse with stress. Lavender essential oil can be applied directly to small area or mixed with a vegetable oil when covering a large area. For an essential oil bath, add fifteen drops of the oil once the bath is already drawn. You can also make a tea using 1 to 2 tsp of flowers; simmer for five minutes in 8 to 16 oz of water, steep for fifteen minutes, and apply or add to a bath.

Licorice is one of the most versatile herbs. It may be used topically for herpes, eczema, ulcers, and canker sores. A tea may be made and the wash may be used topically. Boil 1 tbsp of licorice roots in 8 to 16 oz of water, simmer for fifteen minutes and apply topically as a wash, three times daily. Licorice is also used under professional supervision to help reduce steroid usage (usually standardized tablets with 25 percent glycyrrhic acid are used for this purpose) and for viral infection. People with high blood pressure should not use it internally without professional supervision. However, there is little evidence that less than 3 grams per day will cause blood pressure to rise in healthy people.

Myrrh was used by the ancient Egyptians as an embalming mixture. Today it is usually used for pain syndromes of all sorts, thrush, mouth sores, and ulcer pain. Use tablets or tinctures as directed.

Oats are used topically to stop itching. Oatmeal soap and other products are available at your health food store or pharmacy. You can also make an oatmeal bath by tying a handful of oatmeal into a piece of cotton cloth, and boiling it. Use this as a sponge when you are in the bathtub.

Red Clover is most recently known for its content of flavones, which help women with menopausal symptoms. Traditionally, red clover was used to help people with cancer, and to heal various skin disorders. In England red clover is approved for use in psoriasis, eczema, and rashes. Simmer 1 tbsp in one cup of water for ten minutes and steep for ten minutes; drink three cups per day.

Silica (horsetail)—Silica is necessary for formation of connective tissue. High concentrations are found in the skin and hair, which is why it is used nutritionally to support skin, hair, and bones. It is said to strengthen the skin and reduce wrinkles. In a study where men took silica and fish oil extract, they were able to grow 38 percent more hair.[4] Drink 1 to 3 cups a day of horsetail tea or supplement with 50 mg of silica a day in tablet form. To make a tea, simmer 1 tsp in 8 oz of water for ten minutes; steep five to ten minutes.

Smilax (sarsaparilla) is traditionally used by both Western and Chinese herbalists as a blood purifier. It is typically used for eczema and psoriasis, as well as gouty arthritis. Smilax is an endotoxin binder. Endotoxins are bacterial toxins that aggravate the immune system causing inflammatory reactions such as psoriasis, arthritis, and gout. Simmer 1 to 2 tsp of powdered smilax root in one cup of water for five minutes; steep ten minutes, strain and drink three cups per day.

Witch hazel—This folk remedy is one of the most popular herbs in the U.S., typically used for acne, cuts, bruises, hemorrhoids, and sore muscles. Recently studies have been conducted at the City of Dermatology clinic in Nannheim, Germany, demonstrating the effectiveness of witch hazel cream used with herpes simplex.[5] After eight days, those using witch hazel cream significantly reduced the size and spread of inflammation compared with those in the placebo cream group.

Although the steam distillation water is widely available, herbalists recommend making a decoction of the bark, leaves, and/or twigs as this method appears to bring out the tannins, which contribute the astringent effects of the herb. Boil 1 tsp of powdered roots and twigs in 8 oz of water for ten minutes; strain and cool. Apply directly as a poultice or mix into an ointment.

Skin Formulas

Coptis Purge Fire—This formula is a modification of the traditional formula Long Dan Xie Gan Tang. It is especially useful for acne, rosacea, hives, and dermatitis, where there is redness and inflammation and other eruptions. It is contraindicated when patients have loose stools or diarrhea. It may be used topically as well as internally. Typical dosage is 3 tablets, four times a day. For long term administration, consider combining Coptis Purge Fire (coptis, *huang lian;* lophatherum, *dan zhu ye;* bupleurum, *chai hu;* rehmannia, *sheng di huang; dang gui;* peony, *bai shao;* anemarrhena, *zhi mu;* akebia, *mu tong;* scute, *huang qin;* phellodendron, *huang bai;* alisma, *ze xie;* plantago seed, *che qian zi;* gentiana, *long dan cao;* forsythia, *lian qiao;* gardenia, *zhi zi;* licorice, *gan cao;* sophora, *ku shen)* with Nine Flavor Tea (rehmannia, *shu di huang* and *sheng di huang;* dioscorea, *shan yao;* poria, *fu ling;* cornus, *shan zhu yu;* moutan, *mu dan pi;* alisma, *ze xie;* glehnia, *sha shen;* scrophularia, *xuan shen;* ophiopogon, *mai men dong),* which treats yin deficiency. To make a wash, grind three tablets in a coffee grinder; simmer for five minutes in 16 to 24 oz of water; steep for fifteen minutes; strain; and apply as a wash.

Derma Wind Release (gypsum, *shi gao;* chinese foxglove root, *sheng di huang;* atractylodes rhizome, *cang zhu;* cicada moulting, *chan tui;* tang kuei, *dang gui;* ledebouriella root; siler, *fang feng;* black sesame seeds, *hei zhi ma;* sophora root, *ku shen;* great burdock fruit, *niu bang zi;* schizonepeta, *jing jie;* anemarrhena rhizome, *zhi mu;* licorice root, *gan cao;* akebia caulis, *mu tong)* addresses the interation of Wind-Heat or Wind-Dampness with a preexisting condition of Damp-Heat. It is indicated for weepy, itchy, red skin lesions over a large part of the body, recalcitrant eczema, chronic urticaria, psoriasis, contact dermatitis, Schonlein-Henoch purpura, tinea infection, pruritus, prickly heat, scabies, diaper rash, and skin diseases that become aggravated with hot weather.

Dictamnus 13—This formula is derived from a formula successfully used in England for the treatment of eczema. This formula has traditional herbs to reduce inflammation. Dictamnus (*bai xian pi*), the main herb, has been one of the premier Chinese herbs for treating inflammatory skin conditions when taken internally. It is also used topically for scabies and fungal infections. Other herbs in this formula are synergistic with the principal herb. Dictamnus 13 (dictamnus, *bai xian pi;* siler, *fang feng;* red peony, *chis hao;* tribulus, *bai ji li;* moutan, *mu dan pi;* lophatherum, *dan zhu ye;* rehmannia, *sheng di;* akebia, *mu tong;* sophora, *ku shen;* phellodendron, *huang bai;* atractylodes, *cang zhu;* talc, *hua shi;* licorice, *gan cao*) is a useful formula.

Skin Balance—Designed by master herbalist Fung Fung, this formula has been successfully used with thousands of patients with eczema and psoriasis. It contains traditional anti-inflammatory herbs. It usually takes two to four weeks to see some results; however, major results often take three months or longer. It can be safely taken long term if combined with other herbal formulas. If there is a lot of redness, it may be combined with Clear Heat. If the skin is very dry it is often combined with Marrow Plus. If the patient has weak digestion, it should be combined with digestive remedies such as Six Gentlemen. Reduce the dosage of Skin Balance if loose stools are noticed. General dosage of Skin Balance is two to three tablets three times per day. Skin Balance is comprised of barbat skullcap, *ban zhi lian;* oldenlandia, *bai hua she she cao;* gentian, *long dan cao;* rehmannia root, *sheng di huang;* viola, *zi hua di ding;* siler, *fang feng;* lonicera, *jin yin hua;* lysimachia, *jin qian cao;* coptis root, *huang lian;* tang kuei, *dang gui;* bupleurum, *chai hu;* carthamus (safflower), *hong hua;* senna leaf, *fan xie ye;* and rhubarb, *da huang.*

The Liver Herbs

Burdock (articum, *niu bang zi*)—Burdock is used in both Native American and Chinese herbology. It is used for skin conditions, infections, sciatica, and may have anti-cancer effects. Burdock is considered cooling. It is most appropriate if you have signs of heat such as inflamed skin, fever, constipation, sensations of heat, or anger. It is not appropriate if you have loose stools or cold hands and feet. Typical dosage is 1 tsp of burdock seeds simmered in 8 to 10 oz of water for ten minutes, then steeped for ten minutes. Drink three cups per day.

Ecliptex is a combination of herbs that protect liver function and treat liver damage, as well as hepatitis. It contains eclipta, *han lian cao;* milk thistle, *sylibum marianum;* curcuma, *yu jin;* salvia, *dan shen;* lycium fruit, *gou qi zi;* ligustrum, *nu zhen zi;* bupleurum, *chai hu;* schizandra, *wu wei zi;* tienchi ginseng, *san qi;* tang kuei, *dang gui;* plantago seed, *che qian zi;* licorice, *gan cao.* Typical dosage is three tablets three times per day.

Milk Thistle is usually thought of for its powerful effects at regenerating the liver; however, it is used by herbalists to heal skin conditions, as skin conditions are thought to be a result of faulty detoxification mechanisms. You can either make a tea with milk thistle using the seed, or use extracts which contain 80 percent silymarin. Dosage of tea is 1 to 3 tsp per day; 80 percent silymarin, usually one to four tablets daily (200 to 800 mg a day).

Blood Building Herbs

Herbalists often build up the blood when there are signs of dry or pale skin, itching, history of anemia, or stubborn skin conditions that don't heal. There may also be pale tongue and slow pulse. Tang kuei, also spelled dang gui, is one of the premier blood building herbs. Traditional herbalists never recommend tang kuei by itself. It should always be combined with other herbs. Perhaps the most widely used tang kuei formula is **Eight Treasures** (codonopsis, *dang shen;* atractylodes, *bai zhu;* poria, *fu ling;* rehmannia, *shu di huang;* peony, *bai shao;* red dates, *da zao;* tang kuei, *dang gui;* ligusticum, *chuan xiong;* milletia, *ji xue teng;* baked licorice, *zhi gan cao;* ginger, *gan jiang*). Tang kuei is in the traditional formula Xiao Feng San (XFS), which is indicated for red lesions that are itchy and weepy, and cover a large part of the body.

Marrow Plus (milletia, *ji xue teng;* he shou wu; salvia, *dan shen;* codonopsis, *dang shen;* astragalus, *huang qi;* ligusticum, *chuan xiong;* raw rehmannia, *sheng di huang;* cooked rehmannia, *shu di huang;* lycium, *gou qi zi;* tang kuei, *dang gui;* lotus seed, *lian zi;* citrus, *chen pi;* red date extract, *da zao;* oryza, *gu ya;* gelatinum, *e jiao*) is a modern formula created to strongly tonify blood and increase blood circulation.

Antifungal Herbs

What does antifungal therapy have to do with skin? Many skin conditions involve fungus (athlete's foot, tinea-fungal rash, diaper rash, etc.). Many people find that the drugs are effective temporarily; however, the fungus eventually comes back. Many holistic doctors have found that various other skin conditions such as eczema and psoriasis may also respond to antifungal therapy. Popular herbs for fungal infections include raw garlic, citrus seed extract, which can be either taken as drops or pills, tea tree oil, which is an essential oil that can be applied topically, and pau d'arco, a South American tea which must be consumed at the rate of 6 to 8 cups per day.

Phellostatin helps reduce Candida count naturally and to keep it away. Phellostatin contains phellodendron, *huang bai;* codonopsis, *dang shen;* atractylodes, *bai zhu;* anemarrhena, *zhi mu;* plantago, *che qian zi;* pulsatilla, *bai tou weng;* capillaries, *yin chen hao;* cnidium fruit, *she chuang zi;* houttuynia, *yu xing cao;* dioscorea, *shan yao;* licorice, *gan cao;* cardamon, *sha ren kou.* It may be used with antifungal drugs or other natural therapies. Dosage is 2 to 3 tablets three times a day.

Biocidin (chlorophyll, impatiens pallida, hydrastis canadensis, ferula galbanum, hypericum perforatum, villa rubris, fumaria formosa, frasera carolinensis, gentiana campestris, sanguinaria canadensis, allicin, garlic), is a strong combination of Asian, African, and American herbs.

Oregano oil has been used by nineteenth-century American physicians for pains such as toothache and joint pain and to help grow (nourish) hair. It is an effective antifungal, and can be used topically or internally; add 1 to 3 drops of oregano essential oil to 8 oz of water and take three times a day.

Aromatherapy

Entire books have been written on aromatherapy: the practice of applying essential oils and highly concentrated forms of herbs on the skin, usually with a carrier oil. A good general reference is *The Complete Book of Essential Oils and Aromatherapy* by Valerie Ann Worwood.[6] Below is a list of commonly used essential oils for the skin.

Bergamot	acne
Birch	eczema, ulcers
Carrot	eczema, psoriasis, ulcers
Cedarwood	acne
Chamomile, German	nervous system, acne, dermatitis, eczema, psoriasis, burns
Chamomile, Roman	nervous system, acne, dermatitis
Frankincense	traumatic injury, muscle and joint pain
Galbanum (ferula)	swelling
Geranium	eczema
Grapefruit	obesity, aid in drug withdrawal
Helichrysum	swellings, fungus, bacterial infections
Juniper	obesity, acne, ulcers, swellings
Lavender	acne, boils, burns, inflammation, cuts, wounds, dermatitis, eczema, stress
Lemon	antiseptic, astringent
Lemongrass	insect repellent
Lemon balm	eczema, fungus, bacterial infections, viruses
Tea tree	acne, fungus, wounds, warts, viral infections, bacteria, cold sores, warts, burns, inflammation
Oregano	viral infections, fungus, pain
Patchouli	acne, eczema, skin inflammation, dandruff, insect repellant, antiseptic
Rosemary	skin infections, alopecia (hair loss), obesity, injuries
Sage	sores, bacterial infections, sprains
Sandalwood	acne, fungus and bacteria, skin infections

Tagetes	fungal infections, cuts, sprains, strains, wounds, circulatory problems, antiseptic
Thyme	bacterial infections, viral infections, wounds, immunity-enhancer
Violet	viral and bacterial infections
Yarrow	anti-parasitic, scabies, inflammation

Digestive Support

Many holistic practitioners find it important to heal the digestive system first, as a properly working digestive system helps absorb nutrient and eliminate wastes. In our clinic in Oakland, California, we find many patients with chronic eczema, psoriasis, and hives also have poorly working digestive systems. Combinations that are especially effective include probiotics, such as acidophilus, enzymes that are used to improve food digestion, and Chinese herbal preparations to improve digestion such as Quiet Digestion which contains poria, *fu ling;* coix, *yi yi ren; shen qu;* magnolia, *hou po;* angelica, *bai zhi;* pueraria, *ge gen;* red atractylodes, *cang zhu;* jurinea, *mu xiang;* pogostemon, *huo xiang;* oryza, *gu ya;* trichosanthes root, *tian hua fen;* chrysanthemum, *ju hua;* halloysite, *chi shi zhi;* citrus, *ju hong;* and mentha, *bo he.* Chzyme is a similar preparation with added digestive enzymes.

Constitutional therapies such as Six Gentlemen (codonopsis, *dang shen;* atractylodes, *bai zhu;* poria, *fu ling;* baked licorice, *zhi gan cao;* citrus, *chen pi;* pinellia, *ban xia;* jurinea, *mu xiang;* cardamon, *sha ren)* are used for digestive function and promise long term healing. For more information, see my book, *Healing Digestive Disorders.*

Skin Nutrients

Lipoic acid is one of the premier antioxidants. Because it is both water and fat soluble, it has a wider range of antioxidant activity than vitamins such as C and E. It is a natural compound that exists in each of our bodies, and is also found in liver and yeast. It helps regulate blood sugar, which is why it is recommended for diabetics. In addition, it has anti-inflammatory effects. Topical applications are used to reduce puffiness (edema), redness, enlarged pores, fine lines, and scars. It may be found in health food stores and cosmetic counters, often combined with vitamin C and other antioxidants.

DMAE (dimethylaminoethanol) is an antioxidant stabilizer that helps reduce inflammation. It is naturally found in fish. Although it is best known as an aid to brain function, it is also used to firm up the skin and to treat fine lines above and below the lips. In a study of 17 patients, participants were asked to apply DMAE lotion to one side of the face and neck. After thirty minutes, a difference could be seen between the two halves. DMAE produced an increase in skin tone, producing tighter skin.[7] Topical DMAE products are used by some Hollywood stars for sagging skin, and to make the lips fuller.

Essential fatty acids—Eating fatty fish and taking fish oil, such as cod liver oil, and flax oil are recommended by holistic doctors to reduce the inflammatory response. The treatment of choice for inflammatory skin conditions in remission would be to eat fish (salmon, mackerel, tuna, sardines, herring) three or more times per week. Those clients who have constipation could benefit from taking freshly ground flaxseed (1 to 3 tbsp day) or 1 to 3 tbsp of flax oil. If you use flax oil, it's best to get a brand that must be kept refrigerated and to check the expiration date carefully. If you do not like fish, consider taking a fish oil supplement, containing EPA and DHA. Therapeutic dosage of fish oil is up to 10 g per day with meals. You may also benefit from fish oil if you have fatigue, dry skin, cracked nails, dry hair, constipation, frequent colds, sore joints, or cardiovascular disorders. If you are suffering from active inflammatory outbreak, you might consider a variation on the Swank diet, which has been successfully used with MS and other inflammatory conditions.[8] According to scientists this diet decreases platelet aggregation (i.e., naturally thins your blood), decreases the autoimmune response, increases fatty acid level found in the blood, and increases cerebrospinal fluid. This diet would be especially beneficial for clients with eczema, psoriasis, or scleroderma.

Antioxidant Vitamins—The main antioxidant vitamins are caratenoids, C, E, zinc, and selenium. The antioxidants work best taken together.

Zinc is one of the premier skin nutrients. It is especially useful for acne, mouth ulcers, eczema, and psoriasis. Zinc is also beneficial for the immune system, wound healing, and sexual function, as well as for enhancing vision, taste, and smell. Several double blind studies have shown zinc (citrate or gluconate) has similar results to the antibiotic tetracycline in treating acne.[9] Results are usually seen after

Anti-inflammatory Program

- Consume fish three or more times per week.
- Eat lean meats, poultry, and game, and also use vegetables such as beans and nuts for protein.
- Eliminate margarine, butter, and shortening (these contain unhealthy trans fatty acids that increase inflammatory response).
- Each day use 40 to 50 g (3 to 4 tbsp) of polyunsaturated vegetable oils (avocado, hemp, flax, olive, walnut) as a dressing for salad or cooked vegetables.
- Supplement with at least 1 to 3 tsp of cod liver oil daily.

12 weeks of treatment, and usually dosage is 30 to 50 mg a day. In a study of fifteen patients with contact dermatitis taking 100 mg a day of zinc sulfate, 11 of 15 subjects had complete remission of dermatitis while the other 4 had a 50 to 75 percent reduction of symptoms.[10] However, please note that you should never use over 100 mg of zinc per day.

Carotenes are the reason that vegetables and fruits have vibrant red, yellow, and orange colors. Many holistic physicians are now recommending mixed carotenes containing vitamin A, beta carotene, alpha carotene, and many other beneficial constituents. Carotenes are used for detoxifying, aiding the immune system, improving growth, and reproduction. **Vitamin A** and its derivatives have been used for treatment of acne, psoriasis, ichthyosis, lichen planus, pityriasis rubra pilaris, Darier's disease, and palmoplantar keratoderma. Carotenes, namely beta carotene, have been used for the treatment of photosensitivity disorders and will help protect against sunburn. However, vitamin A by itself should never be used in pregnancy, in amounts greater than 5,000 IU. Signs of vitamin A toxicity include headache, fatigue, muscle and joint pain, and dry skin. Elevated carotene levels do not lead to vitamin A toxicity; however, extremely high dosages of carrot juice, which contains natural carotenoids, can yellow the skin. A beneficial dosage of mixed carotenoids is 10 to 50 mg per day. For good health, eat as many colorful vegetables as possible.

Vitamin C helps us manufacture collagen, the main protein substance of the skin. It helps in the manufacture of nerves and hormones and with utilizing other nutrients. Vitamin C helps fortify the immune system and aids in the detoxification process. It has been clinically used for asthma and other allergies as it appears to lower histamine levels; it is a natural antihistamine. Vitamin C has been clinically used for cancer prevention, heart disease,

Levels of Skin

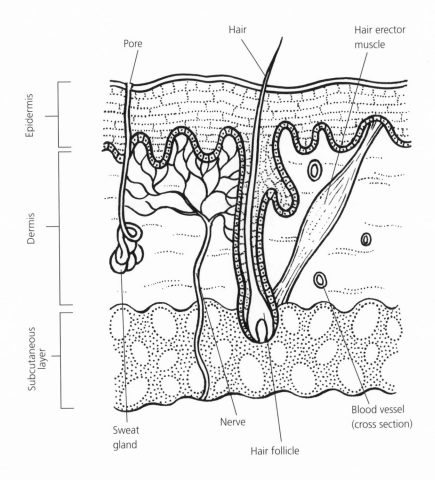

cataracts, common cold, diabetes, complications of pregnancy preelampsia, and premature rupture of fetal membranes. Patients with skin ulcers and bedsores have been shown to have low vitamin C levels. Typical dosage is 1 to 3 grams per day.

Selenium is used to support the immune system and reduce inflammation. Selenium and glutathione levels are low in patients with psoriasis, eczema, and other inflammatory conditions. Typical dosage is 50 to 200 mcg per day. Selenium can also be used topically for viral conditions, such as herpes or shingles. Add a small amount of water to form a paste and cover with gauze. Change dressings two times a day.

Fumaric Acid—Fumaric acid, a chemical naturally occurring in the human body, has been used to treat psoriasis for over thirty years. It appears to alleviate itching and scaling. In several European studies 80 percent of the patients using fumaric acid and a restricted diet noticed good or excellent results.[11] Psoriasis patients are told to avoid pepper, cloves, nutmeg, mustard, caraway seeds, licorice, cinnamon, paprika, luncheon meats, salami, bouillon cubes, mayonnaise, orange, lemon, alcoholic beverages, and nuts. Typical dosage is 500 to 1,000 mg, increased up to 3,000 mg per day over a two-month period (i.e., increasing 500 mg each one to two weeks). Plenty of water should be consumed while taking fumaric acid. Digestive complaints and flushing are noticed by some people, especially those who do not gradually increase their dosage.

Imedeen—Imedeen contains unique proteins from fish. It is used to reduce the visibility of age spots and wrinkles. In a study of 144 patients taking Imedeen for one year, significant improvement was seen in the appearance of fine lines, skin smoothness, and hyper-pigmentation. There were no significant changes noted after only three months.[12] In a ninety-day study of 10 women with sun-damaged skin, those taking Imedeen noticed an improvement in the appearance of wrinkles and dryness of skin. This study was followed up with a thirty-patient trial with similar results.[13] Dosage is 500 mg per day in tablet form.

Chapter Three

Symptoms and Treatments

Acne

Acne occurs when a hair follicle becomes blocked and the skin oil known as *sebum* solidifies and forms a yellowish white plug, thus creating a whitehead. A blackhead is a darkening of the top surface of this plug. When the plug becomes trapped, bacteria in the follicle multiply, irritating the follicle wall. Eventually the follicle ruptures, releasing dead cells and bacteria into the surrounding tissues, leading to inflammation and the typical acne lesion. Three-fourths of teenagers have acne, due to a change in sebum induced by an increase in certain hormones. Acne may be associated with menstrual periods, birth control pills, and stress. Certain medications such as corticosteroids and androgens, which stimulate oil production by the skin, also seem to promote acne. Dermatologists recommend staying away from oily cosmetics and oily sun tan lotions. Seek professional help to remove blackheads. Over-the-counter and prescription medications may be used to promote skin peeling. Tetracycline and other antibiotics may be prescribed, although long-term use may result in systemic yeast infection and other complications. Tretinoin (Retin-A), another prescribed remedy, may cause skin inflammation, scaling, blistering, severe erythema, and pigmentation problems. If you take tretinoin, minimize your exposure to the sun.

While in biomedicine diet is not believed to be a cause of acne, in Chinese medicine it is. Specifically, the pathogenic factors of dampness and heat can lead to acne. Therefore, foods that have a tendency to create dampness and heat should be either reduced or avoided. These include dairy products, chocolate, spicy foods (including chili peppers), sugar and sweets, fried foods, starches, and shellfish. Also, in Chinese medicine, acne is frequently linked to constipation. This is because constipation causes pathogenic factors, such as heat and dampness to accumulate. One of the avenues of elimination is through the skin, thus giving rise to acne.

Lump formation under the skin is known as a *keratinous cyst* or *wen*. A boil-like infection is referred to as *cystic acne*. Both conditions may require local surgery. Washing your face with water only several times a day helps remove excess oil, and may thus reduce the symptoms of keratinous cysts and cystic acne. Dermatologists suggest avoiding iodine, including iodized salt and seaweed (kelp) because the iodine content in these can aggravate acne. Hypoallergenic cosmetics such as those made by the Clinique Company can be very helpful.

Self-Treatments

◆ According to Chinese medicine, to control acne it is essential to eat a diet low in sugar and sweets, alcohol, and dairy products, and to avoid fried foods as much as possible. Other triggers may be soda, chocolate, starches, and shellfish.

- Calendula soap: Calendula is antibacterial. Wash twice daily followed by topical use of witch hazel.
- Zinc: Take 15 to 60 mg daily; add 2 to 3 mg of copper if you take zinc long-term because zinc competes with copper, thus reducing absorption of the latter.
- Tea tree oil: Apply to troubled areas at bedtime, or mix with a clay mask.
- Goldenseal: Follow label directions.
- Acidophilus/bifidus supplement: May be helpful in controlling harmful bacteria. Follow label directions.
- Chromium: Take 200 to 600 mcg daily.

Professional Treatments

- Vitamin A (up to 50,000 IU daily). Vitamin A should be used cautiously during pregnancy; consult your healthcare professional about dosages over 5,000 IU.
- Phellostatin (2 to 3 tablets three times a day): Use to reduce damp-heat, and symptoms of candidiasis due to long-term antibiotic use.
- Nine Flavor Tea (3 tablets three times a day): Use for yin deficiency, including heat-type thirst.
- Coptis Purge Fire: For internal use, take 3 tablets three times a day. For external use, a soak or poultice can be made and applied 1 to 2 times daily. To make a soak, crush 3 tablets; simmer for 5 minutes in 8 to 10 oz water; steep for another 15 minutes, and apply to affected area with a washcloth or cottonball. To make a poultice, crush 3 tablets; mix with a few drops of water until a paste forms; apply to affected area; wash off after 20 minutes.

◆ Resinall K: Especially useful for acne scars. Mix equal parts with witch hazel or hydrogen peroxide, then add a few drops of tea tree oil. Apply 3 times daily.

Case Studies

Case #1

Darla, age fifteen, complained of acne, constant thirst, warts on her toe, and a persistent sore throat. She appeared to have an infection surrounding an eyebrow ring. She was agitated. Traditional Chinese medicine diagnosis revealed that her pulse was racing, and her tongue was red with red spots and patches of yellow coating. From her pulse reading and because her skin felt hot, we suspected that she had a fever. We urged her to see a medical doctor as soon as possible. We also counseled her to drink at least eight glasses of water per day and to give up soda and orange juice because both have high concentrations of sugar, which can lead to an accumulation of damp-heat and thus acne.

She returned two weeks later after having been treated with oral and topical antibiotics for the eyebrow infection. She was weaker and looked paler, and she still had many of the same complaints. Now her pulse was floating and thin, and slightly fast, and her tongue was purplish red and still had red spots; the patches of yellow coating remained. We recommended Nine Flavor Tea (2 tablets four times a day) to replenish yin, and Clear Heat (3 tablets four times a day) to reduce toxicity as evidenced by the acne, warts, and her tongue presentation. She was instructed to reduce the dosage of Clear Heat if she got diarrhea.

By the following week, Darla's symptoms had improved considerably. Her sore throat was gone, her skin was less red, there were fewer signs of acne, and she was no longer thirsty. Her pulse was slower and deeper, and now thin. Her tongue showed fewer red dots and yellow patches. As the acne and warts remained a problem, we suggested she continue drinking 64 oz of water daily and reduce or eliminate greasy foods and sweets, as well as cheese and other dairy foods, which can all lead to damp-heat. To make up the calcium and magnesium she would be lacking from the elimination of dairy products, she was advised to take a multi-mineral formula high in these two elements. We also recommended that she increase the dosage of Nine Flavor Tea (3 tablets three times a day) and reduce the dosage of Clear Heat (1 tablet three times a day). She began cleansing with calendula soap twice daily and washed her skin frequently with water only throughout the day.

After four weeks Darla's skin had improved significantly to the point that she no longer required herbs.

Case #2

Brenda, age seventeen, wore heavy pancake makeup to cover the acne on her face. Traditional Chinese medicine diagnosis revealed that her pulse was wiry and rapid and her tongue was red and dry. We suggested she drink at least 64 oz of water each day, and reduce or eliminate sweets, dairy, and greasy foods. Since she usually drank a few cans of soda or diet soda everyday, we advised her to try stopping. Among other dietary suggestions, we recommended that she take a multivitamin to make up for the calcium and magnesium that she would be missing from eliminating dairy products. In addition, she was given Coptis Purge Fire tincture, to be applied topically at bedtime. Brenda was still wearing heavy makeup, so we urged her to either stop using makeup completely for a few weeks, or to apply as little as possible in order to allow the acne to clear. We also encouraged her to use witch hazel as an antiseptic cleanser. Her next visit one month later revealed an improved skin. Brenda attributed the change to faithfully carrying out all our instructions.

Discussion: Teenage acne can be very difficult to treat because clients are often not willing to give up sweets, dairy products, and foods that are high in fats. Therefore, in addition to recommending internal and topical herbs, and using hypoallergenic cosmetics, counseling about diet, cosmetic usage, and skin care are necessary components of the overall treatment protocol.

Case #3

Laverne, thirty-five, complained of facial acne. She was under a great deal of stress and suffered from constipation. Traditional Chinese medicine diagnosis revealed that her pulse was wiry and rapid and her tongue had a heavy gray-yellow coating.

We first suggested Laverne give up soda and drink at least 64 oz of water daily, and that she minimize or eliminate alcohol, greasy foods, and dairy products from her diet. We also recommended that she increase her consumption of greens and other vegetables, and that she switch to hypoallergenic cosmetics. She was given the formulas Calm Spirit (3 tablets three times a day) to help decrease stress and nourish yin, and Coptis Purge Fire (2 tablets three times a day) for its antibacterial effects and to reduce damp-heat. A multimineral supplement was used to make up for the lost calcium and magnesium from her stopping dairy products. After three weeks Laverne's skin had improved greatly. In addition, she felt calmer. Her bowel function had also improved—she was now having a bowel movement every day.

Case #4

Theresa, a twenty-year-old student, had been taking tetracyline for two years to treat her acne and wanted to discontinue it. Traditional Chinese medicine diagnosis revealed that her pulse was wiry and her tongue had a yellow-gray coating.

We recommended the formula Coptis Purge Fire (3 tablets three times a day). We also suggested she make a wash with Coptis Purge Fire by crushing 2 tablets, simmering in 8 oz of water for five minutes, and steeping for another fifteen minutes, then straining. We instructed her to use the herbal wash twice daily, followed by witch hazel, on the face and other affected areas. In addition, she was counseled about decreasing or eliminating alcohol, sweets, dairy products, fried foods, and junk food. Other diet recommendations included increasing her water and fresh vegetable intake, and taking 50,000 IU of vitamin A per day, as well as a multimineral supplement.

After one week Theresa developed diarrhea, so we suggested reducing the Coptis Purge Fire to 2 tablets three times a day. We also recommended Colostroplex (1 tablet three times a day), to treat diarrhea and heal the intestines, which were probably damaged by the extensive use of antibiotics; Colostroplex appears to restore the natural gastrointestinal flora. We also recommended she eat a porridge made of pearl barley every morning since traditional Chinese medicine uses pearl barley to eliminate dampness and nourish the skin. Two weeks later, Theresa showed slight improvement. But a few days before her next appointment she developed a bad outbreak on her face and was afraid she would have to resume taking the antibiotics. Her pulse was now slow and slightly wiry, and her tongue coating was less thick. Upon query she stated that she had not been applying the Coptis Purge Fire wash. We again urged her to use the wash, and follow it with witch hazel. We also suggested she continue the herbs and Colostroplex as above.

After two weeks Theresa reported no outbreaks except after eating chocolate. Overall her skin appeared less oily; however, her face had acne scars and visible purplish vessels. At this point, she mentioned that she got frequent vaginal yeast infections. We adjusted her protocol to treat for fungus, as we suspected the prolonged antibiotic use had caused a systemic proliferation of yeast. Her pulse was wiry and her tongue was pale with swollen edges, and had a gray coating in the rear. We recommended Skin Balance (1 tablet three times a day), Colostroplex (1 tablet three times a day), and Phellostatin (2 tablets three times a day). Phellostatin contains herbs with antifungal properties as well as tonic herbs to aid the digestive system. She continued using the Coptis Purge Fire wash and witch hazel. We also had her wash her face daily with calendula soap.

Over the next three months Theresa took the herbs and supplements as directed. She also noticed that her acne outbreaks were directly related to her consumption of chocolate and other sweets, fried foods, and beer, which prompted her to be more vigilant about what she ate. A face peel from a dermatologist eliminated some of the scars from previous outbreaks.

Case #5

Claire, twenty-four, a secretary, had recently had a breakout of acne. When she came to our clinic she was taking tetracyline to control the acne. She also had a history of vaginal yeast infections, frequent colds and flu, and chronic constipation. Traditional Chinese medicine diagnosis revealed that her pulse was rapid and her tongue was bright red.

We first urged her to eliminate alcohol, sweets, dairy products, and fried foods from her diet. We also recommended a combination of Aquilaria 22 (2 tablets three times a day) and Phellostatin (1 tablet three times a day the first week, 2 tablets three times a day in the second week). In addition, we suggested she drink at least eight glasses of water each day and that she use witch hazel topically after washing her face.

After two weeks Claire felt her acne had improved slightly. Her constipation was also better, as she was now having bowel movements every other day instead of just twice a week. Her pulse was still rapid and her tongue bright red, so she was asked to increase the dose of Aquilaria 22 (to 3 tablets three times a day) and continue taking Phellostatin (2 tablets three times a day). Finally, we suggested she wash with Coptis Purge Fire (2 tablets crushed and simmered in 8 oz water for five minutes, steeped for fifteen minutes, and then strained) and applied twice per day. After three weeks, Claire's skin had improved nearly ninety percent. Her constipation was also much better, as she was now having daily bowel movements.

Case #6

Kristen, a thirty-one-year-old housewife, complained of acne, PMS symptoms, menstrual cramps, insomnia, and constipation. She was a smoker, and indulged in a diet high in both fat and sugar. Traditional Chinese medicine diagnosis revealed that her pulse was weak and slightly rapid, and her tongue was purple and dry.

We first recommended a modified anti-yeast diet, and suggested she take Woman's Balance (2 tablets three times a day) and Coptis Purge Fire (2 tablets three times a day). We also encouraged her to use a Coptis Purge Fire wash twice per day (see previous case for instructions) and that she wash her face with calendula soap followed by witch hazel twice daily also. After two weeks Kristen's acne looked less red; however, she was still constipated, suggesting there was still excess heat trapped in her body and contributing to the acne. Her pulse and tongue were unchanged as well. She was asked to increase the dosage of Coptis Purge Fire (to 3 tablets three times a day to remove damp-heat) and continue taking Woman's Balance (2 tablets three times a day) to move liver qi and reduce heat. Three weeks later, her acne showed continued improvement. It had not flared up pre-menstrually, as was normally the case, and she was less constipated. At this point, we advised Kristen to reduce or eliminate sweets, dairy products, coffee, fried foods, and alcohol, so that the damp-heat would be held in check. We also referred her to a colleague for ear acupuncture to help her quit smoking. Although she was only able to stop completely for three days, Kristen did reduce her smoking from half a pack to three cigarettes per day. She also felt the acupuncture was helpful for stress reduction. Kristen kept taking the herbs for another three months, and all symptoms gradually improved. If she continues with herbal therapy, we will recommend supplementing with the formula Nine Flavor Tea to nourish yin and reduce deficiency heat to help control her acne.

Case #7

Frank, a twenty-nine-year-old sales professional, had recently had an outbreak of acne. He had been on antibiotics throughout his teens to control acne and was anxious to try a more natural approach. He indicated that he usually had a few drinks after work and that because he is single and does not cook, he eats most of his meals at restaurants. Traditional Chinese medicine diagnosis revealed that his pulse was rapid and his tongue had a thin yellow-gray coating.

We advised him to eliminate or greatly reduce alcohol, improve his diet, increase his water intake to 64 oz per day, and eliminate his usual beverages of coffee and fruit juice, both of which can give rise to damp-heat and thus acne. We also recommended he clean his face with calendula soap twice a day and apply witch hazel afterwards. Additionally, he was asked to use hypoallergenic products (such as shaving cream) since the standard commercial products often contain allergens. The supplements we recommended were Coptis Purge Fire (3 tablets three times a day), vitamin A (50,000 IU per day), and a broad-spectrum, antioxidant formula containing zinc.

During his next visit two weeks later, we saw that Frank's acne had worsened with more lesions on the face and more frequent outbreaks. He said he had tried to cut down on alcohol, but had experienced an increased craving for sweets, especially chocolate, which he knew was a problematic food for him. He had not been able to purchase some of the items we had recommended, such as the vitamin A, calendula soap, and hypoallergenic shaving cream. His pulse was rapid and irregular, and his tongue was purple, although the coating was less thick. We urged him to buy the items we had recommended, and to try to plan his schedule so that he could get in some exercise after work rather than going out drinking.

A month later, Frank's acne had improved. He had followed all our suggestions, including limiting his alcohol intake to one night a week. His pulse was slower, and his tongue coating was more normal. After another month, he had no further outbreaks, and his skin looked much healthier than when he first came in. He will soon begin a trial period off the herbs and will begin tapering off the vitamin A. He indicated that he would continue to follow the diet and other recommendations.

Age Spots

Age spots, also known as liver spots, are flat patches of increased pigmentation that result as a buildup of waste material in the skin. They range in size from a freckle to a few inches. Medical doctors sometimes prescribe Retin-A for age spots. Herbalists say that contributing factors to age spots are poor liver function, poor diet, and excessive sun exposure. Avoiding smoking and excessive sun exposure, eating plenty of fresh fruits and vegetables, and drinking at least 64 oz of fluid in the form of water or herbal tea will help to preserve your skin.

Self-Treatments

◆ Broad-spectrum antioxidant formula (follow label instructions).
◆ Vitamin E (400 to 800 IU) daily.
◆ Grape seed extract or pycnogenol (50 mg three times a day).
◆ Imedeen biomarine supplements (follow label instructions).
◆ Hydroquinone (active ingredient in skin bleaching products such as Brown Spot Skin Lightening Night Cream manufactured by Reviva; follow label instructions).
◆ Vitamin C topically (follow label instructions).
◆ Alpha lipoic acid topically (follow label instructions).

Athlete's Foot

Athlete's foot is a fungal infection known medically as *tinea pedis.* As fungus generally grows in dark, moist environments, athlete's foot is associated with sweating and wearing shoes. Methods for controlling and preventing athlete's foot include walking barefoot while in clean, dry surroundings, wearing white, breathable socks that can be changed at least once a day, and cleaning the feet—especially between the toes—one or more times daily. After each cleaning, dry your feet well; using a blow dryer will help remove moisture. In addition, wearing thongs in locker rooms and showers is one important way to protect yourself from cross-infection. Disinfecting shower floors also helps control the spread of athlete's foot. If you already have this condition, over-the-counter lotions, sprays, and powders may be found at health food or drugstores. Lamisil lotion is particularly effective; use as directed.

Self-Treatments

♦ Licorice foot soak: Licorice contains natural antifungal compounds that can be helpful in treating athlete's foot. To make a soak, add 4 teaspoons of dried licorice to 1 cup of water. Bring to boil and simmer for 20 minutes. Add to a large basin, containing 1 quart of lukewarm water. Add 12 drops of oregano oil, tea tree oil, or citrus seed extract. Soak feet for 10 minutes, 1 to 2 times daily. Dry thoroughly.

♦ Wash feet well with calendula soap 1 to 2 times daily. Apply tea tree oil topically afterwards: 1 part tea tree oil to 2 parts hot water.

Professional Treatments

♦ Anti-yeast protocol. (See Anti-fungal herb section.)

♦ Clear Heat foot soak: To make a soak, crush 3 tablets; simmer for 5 minutes in 8 to 10 oz water; steep for another 15 minutes; add to a large basin containing 1 quart of lukewarm water. Soak feet for 10 minutes, 1 to 2 times daily. Dry thoroughly. Add essential oils or Biocidin if desired.

♦ Resinall K: Apply to affected area 1 to 2 times daily.

♦ Biocidin: Add 5 drops to a large basin containing 1 quart of hot water. Soak feet for 15 minutes, 1 to 2 times daily.

Case Study

Keith, a twenty-three-year-old athlete, had chronic athlete's foot. He also had nail fungus of the toes, recurrent jock itch, and tinea versicolor that affected his torso. Although he had been prescribed antifungal medication, the fungus kept recurring. Keith was concerned that the medication was harmful to his liver. Therefore, he came to our clinic seeking a natural approach to his problems. Traditional Chinese medicine diagnosis revealed that his pulse was fast and wiry, and his tongue was reddish purple.

We suggested he try the formula Phellostatin (2 tablets three times a day) along with Biocidin (1 to 4 drops with meals). In addition to using these two remedies internally, we recommended that he use the Biocidin as a soak for his feet, and as a wash for his groin and torso (3 drops Biocidin added to 1 quart of hot water—three-quarters used for the soak, and one-quarter used for the wash). Finally, we urged Keith to incorporate an anti-yeast diet. After three months, he had no signs of fungal infection except the tinea on his torso. We continued trying various natural remedies, which helped improve the condition, but none were able to completely resolve the tinea. In the end, he had to resort to topical Nizoral to control the infection on his torso.

Boils (Furuncles) and Carbuncles

A boil is an infection of a hair follicle by the bacteria *Staphylococcus*. The result is formation of a swollen, tender, pink or red nodule with a yellowish tip. Occasionally, a boil will go away without treatment. Usually, however, it will grow over a period of a few days, filling with pus and causing increasing pain. Eventually, some boils burst, drain, and heal. If a boil bursts, great care needs to be taken to prevent the infection from spreading and to keep the open wound clean. Boils most often occur on the face, neck, armpits, buttocks, or thighs. If a boil lasts more than ten days, or is located on the spine or face, see a physician immediately. It is also important to see a health professional for furunculosis (frequently recurring boils). Boils on the face or spine, or frequently recurring boils, may lead to serious conditions such as brain or spinal abscesses, or life-threatening infections.

Recently developed boils not on the face may be treated with warm water compresses applied for as long as possible to relieve discomfort and promote drainage. Frequent Epsom salt baths may also be helpful. It is particularly important to wash the infected area frequently with antibacterial soap. Do not squeeze or puncture the boil, as this may spread the infection. Physicians may recommend antibiotics or may drain the boil surgically.

A carbuncle is a cluster of boils caused by the spreading of the staph infection beneath the skin. Carbuncles usually appear on the neck and upper back, and may be accompanied by pain, fever, and fatigue. Boils and carbuncles are associated with poor hygiene, acne, dermatitis, diabetes, anemia, and decreased immune function. They can also occur when one is generally rundown or under stress. Both boils and carbuncles may be spread from person to person; therefore, hygiene measures such as frequent handwashing are important in preventing the spread.

Self-Treatments

- According to Chinese medicine, boils and carbuncles are often due to accumulated heat. Therefore, limit alcohol, sweets, greasy foods, and coffee since these can give rise to heat.
- Broad-spectrum antioxidants (follow label directions).
- Vitamin C (1,000 mg daily).

- Vitamin A (10,000 to 25,000 IU daily). High dosages of vit-
  amin A should not be taken by pregnant women.
- Iron and zinc, if deficient. Deficiency is determined through
  blood tests.
- Vitamin E topically during the healing stages (2 times daily).
- Goldenseal tincture: Apply topically (3 times daily) after thor-
  oughly washing the area.
- Calendula soap (3 times daily).

Professional Treatments

- Clear Heat: For internal use, take 3 tablets three times a day;
  for external use, crush 3 tablets; simmer in 16 oz water for
  15 minutes; strain and apply with washcloth (3 times daily).
- Resinall K: Apply directly on affected area (2 times daily).
- Proteolytic enzymes such as bromelain (2,000 mg daily): Use
  to reduce swelling.
- Coptis Purge Fire (3 tablets three times a day): Use for damp-
  heat pattern.
- Nine Flavor Tea (3 tablets three times a day): Use for yin deficiency pattern.
- Coptis Purge Fire wash: Crush 2 tablets; simmer in 8 oz of
  water for five minutes; steep for another fifteen minutes, then
  strain. Use washcloth to apply 2 to 3 times daily.

Bruising

Bruising is often a result of increased fragility of the blood vessels. It is commonly seen in seniors and can also be a sign of serious disease. If you notice increased bruising that is not associated
with minor trauma, it is important to see a health professional

since bruising may be associated with medical conditions such as anemia, platelet disorders (such as idiopathic thrombocytopenic purpura or ITP), liver damage, cancer, lupus, and accumulated copper.

Self-Treatments

- Vitamin E (400 to 800 IU daily).
- Proteolytic enzymes such as bromelain (1,000 mg daily).
- St. John's wort oil: Apply topically (2 to 3 times daily).

Professional Treatments

- Comfrey poultice: Mix 1 tsp of powder with water; add water using a dropper to make a paste. Apply 2 to 3 times daily. Do not apply to an open wound.
- Resinall E: Take following trauma (3 tablets daily until bruise heals).
- Resinall K: Use topically following trauma. Dilute 1 part Resinall K with 1 part rubbing alcohol, apply one-half dropper three times a day, and massage into the bruised area 5 to 6 times daily.
- For a tendency to bruise easily use Marrow Plus (3 tablets three times a day) to tonify the blood and treat anemia; and Enhance (3 tablets four times a day) to help boost platelet counts, especially for individuals with idiopathic thrombocytopenic purpura (ITP).

Bunions

A bunion is a protrusion at the base of the big toe. Although genetics predispose some people to bunions, bunions are often caused by wearing high heels or shoes with pointed toes. To avoid bunions and the pain they cause, wear flatter and more comfortable shoes or sandals, or go barefoot whenever possible. Felt pads (mole skins) are available in pharmacies and can be applied over bunions. Orthotics (shoe inserts) can be custom-made by a podiatrist to relieve discomfort.

Self-Treatments

- Clove essential oil: Apply to the bunion directly several times daily.
- Capsaicin cream or ointment: Capsaicin is the active ingredient in chili peppers and is effective against pain.
- White flower oil: Contains wintergreen oil, which is effective against pain.

Foot Care

- Wear shoes that fit. Corns and calluses occur as a result of wearing shoes that are too tight or too loose.
- Wear breathable footwear, such as leather or canvas.
- Wear white cotton socks, because they absorb sweat.
- To remove calluses, use a pumice stone.
- To prevent dry skin, apply a foot cream at night.
- To control athlete's foot, mix 5 drops tea tree oil per 1 tsp water. Put in spray bottle and spray foot several times daily. Or, use commercial tea tree oil products available in health food stores (follow label directions).
- A foot bath is a great way to relax the feet. Adding an essential oil can help soften the skin and reduce fungal growth. Suitable oils include tea tree, orange, rose, geranium, cedarwood, and lavender.

- Arnica ointment: Apply directly to the bunion (follow label directions).
- Turmeric tea: Turmeric has anti-inflammatory properties. Combine one-half tsp of powder in 8 oz hot water (take 1 to 3 times daily).

Professional Treatments

- Resinall E (3 tablets either three or four times a day).
- Resinall K: For internal use, take one-half dropperful three times a day; for topical use, apply one-half dropperful four times a day to the bunion.

Burns

A first-degree burn affects only the outer layer of skin, known as the *epidermis,* and is marked by redness, swelling, and pain. A second-degree burn affects the second layer of skin, known as the *dermis,* and is characterized by very red skin, severe swelling and pain, and the development of blisters. A third-degree burn is the most serious, affecting all skin layers, and is marked by skin that appears either white or charred black. Third-degree burns can injure the nerves, muscles, and bones, as well as the skin.

Seek medical assistance (call 911) for first-degree burns larger in area than six inches, for second-degree burns affecting the hands, feet, face, groin, or buttocks, and for all third-degree burns. Likewise, electrical and chemical burns can be very serious and require immediate medical attention. For less severe burns, run cold water over the area or submerge it in cool water. Aspirin, ibuprofen, or other analgesics and nonsteroidal anti-inflammatory medications (NSAIDs) can be administered to relieve pain and reduce swelling.

Self-Treatment

♦ Aloe vera: Apply juice or lotion topically. To speed healing, mix with 4 drops lavender essential oil and apply to affected area or place a moist peppermint tea bag over the affected area.

Professional Treatments

Use the following in addition to the treatments mentioned above:

♦ Astra C (2 to 3 tablets three times a day): Use to help regenerate skin.
♦ Resinall K: Use to help speed healing (1 part Resinall K to 3 parts safflower oil; apply 3 times daily).

Case Study

Nick, nine-years-old, came to our clinic immediately after burning his hand on a hot water pipe. His hand was very red and was starting to swell. We mixed one part Resinall K with four parts water. He took the remedy home and applied it to the burn with a cloth for thirty minutes. He continued to use the Resinall K over the next three days, applying it three times daily. We also asked him to take Astra C (2 tablets three times a day) to speed healing. In a follow-up telephone call three days after his visit, Nick indicated that the pain and swelling were gone, and his skin was no longer so red.

Canker Sores

Canker sores are known biomedically as aphthous ulcers, which are a very common form of mouth ulcer. More women than men develop them. Biomedically, the cause is not known. There may be a genetic predisposition to developing canker sores, or it may be some kind of immune response. Triggers include injury to the oral mucosal lining from dental procedures and from bites. Stress, menstruation, food allergies, as well as dietary deficiencies such as vitamin B12, folic acid, or iron, are also linked to canker sore development.

Biomedically, canker sores are not treated because they usually resolve spontaneously in one to three weeks. More severe cases should be evaluated to rule out other causes such as acute herpes simplex, erythema multiforme, pemphigus, among other disorders.

Self-Treatments

- Clove essential oil: Use to heal an active sore. Dab with a cotton swab on the sore several times daily, holding the swab against the sore for a minute or two.
- Myrrh tincture: Use on active sore. Apply in same manner as clove oil.
- Zinc lozenges: Speed healing and promotes the immune system (follow label directions).
- Acidophilus/bifidus (2 capsules or one-half teaspoon three times a day). Use to help prevent canker sores.
- B-complex vitamin and folic acid supplements: Use to help prevent canker sores (follow label directions).

Professional Treatments

◆ Coptis Purge Fire (3 tablets, 4 to 6 times daily): Use to help reduce severity of flare-ups. Reduce dosage if diarrhea occurs.

◆ Isatis Gold (3 capsules or tablets four times a day): Contains goldenseal, echinacea, and isatis, which help reduce swelling, dispel heat toxin, and promote blood flow.

◆ Resinall K: Use to help relieve pain. Soak a cotton swab in one-half dropperful Resinall K. Hold swab on the sore for 1 to 2 minutes. (Apply 3 to 4 times daily.)

◆ Clearing (3 tablets four times a day): Use for signs of stomach yin deficiency. Stomach yin deficiency is characterized by fever or feeling hot in the afternoon, dry mouth and throat, thirst, and feeling excessively full after eating. This formula is used as a preventive.

◆ If blood tests reveal anemia, consider supplementation with Marrow Plus (3 tablets three times a day).

Case Studies

Case #1

Neil, a forty-nine-year-old contractor, was previously treated successfully at our clinic for ulcerative colitis. He now presented with recurrent canker sores and eczema, especially behind the ears and on the scalp and hands. He also complained of fatigue and sensitivity to the sun. Whenever he was in the sun for a long period, his skin was extremely itchy and he often broke out in hives. Traditional Chinese medicine diagnosis revealed that his pulse was rapid, and his tongue was red with a thick yellow coating.

We recommended that for the next three months he resume taking Colostroplex (1 to 2 tablets two times a day), and Quercenol (2 tablets two times a day with meals). These two formulas had been very effective in addressing Neil's colitis problems. Colostroplex is a formula that helps rid the body of bacteria, viruses, and fungus, and restores gastrointestinal immunity. Quercenol is an antioxidant formula. Holistic practitioners believe antioxidants reduce the inflammatory response. Quercenol also contains quercetin, which may help reduce allergy, and zinc, which promotes skin health. Finally, we recommended that if canker sores recurred, Neil use Coptis Purge Fire (3 tablets 4 to 6 times per day, to be reduced if loose stools occur).

We discussed having Neil again restrict his intake of wheat, alcohol, dairy, sweets, and corn, which had helped alleviate the colitis symptoms. Particular triggers for him were creamy soups and dressings, corn, and chocolate. The other items he could consume on an occasional basis.

One week later, the canker sores were gone. At this point, Neil's pulse was less rapid, and tongue coating less thick. We suggested that he continue on the Colostroplex and Quercenol at the same dosages, and take Skin Balance (2 tablets three times a day). Two weeks later, he reported that the eczema was improved; however, he was having loose stools. His pulse was normal, and although his tongue still had a yellow coating, it was not as thick. As a result, we added Six Gentlemen (3 tablets four times a day), which tonifies the spleen, and suggested he reduce the Skin Balance (1 tablet four times a day) and continue with the Colostroplex and Quercenol. We tried Resinall K topically for the lesions on his hands and behind his ears. As his scalp continued to itch, we suggested he shampoo his hair every other day, and rinse it with water alone on the alternate days.

After two weeks, Neil felt the Resinall K had reduced the itching on his hands and behind his ears; however, his scalp still itched. His pulse was slightly wiry, and his tongue coating was about the same. We asked him if he was watching what he ate, and he replied that he had been under a lot of stress and was not able to make the suggested changes. We encouraged him to do his best. He remained on the herbal protocol, and to address the scalp itching, we suggested an over-the-counter anti-itch shampoo.

Neil continued herbal therapy for the next two months. He had great faith in the herbs, as they had previously enabled him to stop the prednisone, which he had depended on to control his colitis. At this point his eczema, loose stools, and canker sores were able to be managed through diet and using herbs.

Case #2

Joyce, a fifty-four-year-old secretary, had chronic canker sores since she was a young girl. The sores recurred once or twice a month, and typically lasted up to two weeks. She was also experiencing menopausal symptoms. Traditional Chinese medicine diagnosis revealed that her pulse was thin and rapid, and her tongue was pale, dry, and swollen.

As she was currently suffering from canker sores, we suggested she take Coptis Purge Fire (3 tablets 4 to 6 times per day, to be reduced if loose stools occurred). We also recommended applying Resinall K by dipping a cotton swab in half a dropperful of the formula, and then holding in contact with the sores for one to two minutes (4 to 6 times per day). She called back three days later to say that the sores were gone, which was the fastest they had ever disappeared.

Joyce's next visit was one week later. We recommended she try Astra Isatis and Calm Spirit (2 tablets of each formula four times a day) to prevent the canker sores from recurring. Astra Isatis is used to strengthen the immune system and to clear heat.

Calm Spirit helps relieve stress and nourishes the yin. Over the next six months, Joyce remained on this preventive protocol, switching to Coptis Purge Fire and Resinall K twice when a canker sore recurred. She was also advised to avoid spicy foods, acidic foods, alcohol, and other foods and beverages that provoke heat and can cause canker sores.

Case #3

Mary, a forty-five-year-old executive assistant, complained of canker sores, low grade fever, abdominal cramping, constipation, and burning sensation upon passing of stools. Traditional Chinese medicine diagnosis revealed that her pulse was rapid, and her tongue was red with a yellow coating.

We recommended Coptis Purge Fire (3 tablets 4 to 6 times per day, to be reduced if loose stools occur). We also had her use Resinall K, which was applied by dipping a cotton swab in half a dropperful of the formula, then holding it in contact with the sores for one to two minutes (4 to 6 times per day). After one week the canker sores were reduced, the fever was gone, and her constipation was relieved. Her pulse was less rapid and her tongue showed less coating. However, Mary still had abdominal cramping, most likely from a poor diet and stress. At this point, we suggested she continue to use Resinall K as directed, and that she substitute Isatis Cooling (3 tablets four times a day) for Coptis Purge Fire. We also suggested she take PB-8 acidophilus, 2 capsules before bed and 2 capsules on an empty stomach during the day.

After two weeks the canker sores were resolved, with a reduction or elimination of all other symptoms. Mary's pulse was now normal and her tongue no longer had a yellow coating. We therefore recommended she take Clearing (3 tablets four times a day), and PB-8 acidophilus (2 capsules two times a day) on an empty stomach for the next several months. We also counseled her against eating spicy foods, alcohol, and dairy products, with the exception of homemade yogurt, which contains beneficial acidophilus.

Discussion: Coptis Purge Fire was initially recommended to clear heat and dampness. Resinall K was used topically, as we have found through experience at our clinic that the formula reduces canker sores and has pain-relieving properties. After one week, we switched Mary to Isatis Cooling since this formula is more specific for abdominal pain, although it also has heat-clearing actions. PB-8 acidophilus was used as a long-term preventive aid for canker sores, as was Clearing, which has properties that nourish the yin, clear heat, and reduce dampness. Clearing is a tonic and is more appropriate than Isatis Cooling or Coptis Purge Fire for long-term administration when heat signs are not as prominent.

Cellulite

Cellulite is lumpy fat usually found in the thighs, hips, and buttocks of women. It can cause pitting, bulging, and deformation of the skin around it, as well as tightness, heaviness, or tenderness. The standard recommended treatment is weight loss. The most effective programs emphasize gradual weight loss, regular exercise, eating lean protein, increasing fresh fruits and vegetables in the diet, and drinking 64 oz of water per day. Rapid weight loss can actually make cellulite-related pitting and bulging more apparent. While liposuction can be used to remove fat, there are many potential side effects including bleeding, infection, and injury to the veins, nerves, and arteries that supply the skin.

Self -Treatments

- Bladderwrack: This type of seaweed helps induce weight loss, perhaps due to its high iodine content, which may promote thyroid function, and thus metabolism. Use 1 tsp stirred into 8 oz water (take 1 to 3 times daily). It is also an empirical topical treatment for cellulite. Mix 1 tsp in 8 oz water. Massage into the affected area with the hand or a soft brush (3 times daily).
- Gotu kola (at least 4,500 mg daily): Appears to firm the connective tissue.

Professional Treatments

- Drain Dampness (3 tablets three times a day): Use to help reduce edema.
- Astra 18 (3 tablets, half an hour before each meal): Use to promote healthy weight loss. This formula has phlegm-reducing and some diuretic actions.
- Astra Diet Tea (3 cups per day): Pleasant tasting substitute for sweets, also helps boost energy.
- Flavonex (3 tablets three times a day): Use to promote circulation so as to reduce cellulite.
- Resinall K: For internal use, take one-half dropperful three times a day to help repair and restore the skin; for external use, mix 1 part Resinall K with 1 part safflower oil, then massage twice daily into the skin to help resolve pitting.

Chickenpox (varicella)

Chickenpox is a highly contagious disease that is mild in children, but can be quite serious in adults. It is marked by a clearly recognizable rash, as well as fever and fatigue. The rash begins as small, red, itchy spots. Within a few hours the spots transform into blisters filled with clear fluid; after several days the blisters dry and scab.

Those afflicted with chickenpox are highly infectious from approximately two days before the appearance of the rash to a week later. During this period adults who have never had chickenpox should avoid contact with those afflicted. Cool compresses may help relieve the itching, and frequent baths will help prevent infections. In addition, keeping children's nails short and clean can prevent secondary bacterial infection and scarring from scratching.

Biomedical treatment sometimes involves the use of antihistamines to relieve itching. The antiviral medication, Acyclovir, is prescribed for severe infections involving the lungs or brain. Complications of chickenpox, such as pneumonia, are treated with antibiotics. The varicella vaccine is now available for routine immunization.

Self-Treatments

♦ Vitamin A (20,000 to 50,000 IU daily for adults; for children, use one-quarter the adult dosage): stimulates the immune system and aids in the healing of skin and tissue. One of the best natural sources of vitamin A is fish oil. Vitamin A should be used cautiously during pregnancy; consult your health-care professional about dosages over 5,000 IU.

- Red clover wash: Steep 1 tsp in 8 oz hot water for 20 minutes. Apply 3 times daily.
- Goldenseal: Use internally as directed on the package; use tincture externally by dabbing on the lesions with a cotton swab 3 times daily.
- Witch hazel: Use cotton swab to dab lesions 4 to 6 times daily.
- Chamomile cream: Apply to the lesions 3 times daily.

Professional Treatments

The following formulas are typically combined as Clear Heat is more effective at reducing itching, whereas Coptis Purge Fire is better for healing blisters.

- Clear Heat: For internal use, adults take 2 tablets, 4 to 6 times daily; children take 1 tablet per 10 pounds of body weight daily. For external use, crush 3 tablets; add to 8 oz boiling water; steep for 10 to 15 minutes; and apply fluid as a cool or lukewarm compress to relieve itching.
- Coptis Purge Fire: Adults take 2 tablets, 4 to 6 times daily; children take 1 tablet per 10 pounds of body weight daily.

Case Study (Adult Chickenpox)

Lydia, thirty-five, had contracted adult chickenpox, and experienced the characteristic itchy rash. She also had been running a 102°F fever for several days. Her medical doctor said there was little to do other than drink plenty of fluids, apply cool water compresses, and take antihistamines for the itching and Tylenol for the fever. When she came to our clinic, traditional Chinese medicine diagnosis revealed that her pulse was rapid, and her tongue was red with a yellow coating.

We recommended Coptis Purge Fire and Clear Heat (2 tablets of each formula 4 to 6 times daily). A few days later, Lydia's fever had dropped to 99°F. She also felt the herbs had helped reduce the itching.

Cold Sores (Herpes Simplex)

There are two main kinds of herpes simplex virus: type 2 is transmitted sexually and causes genital herpes (see section later in this chapter); type 1 causes cold sores (also known as fever blisters), and is contracted through kissing, or by sharing food, kitchen utensils, towels, or razors with an infected family member or another individual. Cold sores are most likely to occur on or around the mouth, lips, and gums, where small fluid-filled blisters may arise from red painful areas of skin. Outbreaks range from mild to quite painful and may last one week or longer. Stress, fever, sun exposure, and menstruation may trigger recurrence. To inhibit the ability of the herpes virus to replicate, holistic practitioners often recommend increasing the amino acid lysine and decreasing the amino acid arginine.[14] Lysine-rich foods include fish, chicken, cheese, beef, beans, brewer's yeast, mung bean sprouts, and most fruits and vegetables. Avoid chocolate, carob, coconut, oats, flour, bread, peanuts, soybeans, and wheat germ because these contain arginine.

Self-Treatments

- Vitamin C (1,000 mg daily).
- Lysine (1,200 mg).
- Lemon balm wash: Boil 1 tsp dried lemon balm in 8 oz water for 5 minutes, steep for 15 minutes, and apply the fluid 4 to 6 times daily.

- Broad-spectrum antioxidant for prevention (follow label instructions).
- St. John's wort topically: Apply the oil or salve form 4 to 6 times daily.

Professional Treatments

- Coptis Purge Fire (3 tablets, 4 to 6 times per day): Use to treat cold sores. (Reduce dosage if diarrhea occurs.)
- Astra Isatis (2 to 3 tablets three times a day): Use to prevent cold sores and to tonify the immune system.
  - For heat signs, add Clear Heat (2 to 3 tablets three times a day).
  - For cold signs, add Power Mushroom (1 to 2 tablets three times a day).
- Resinall K: Soak a cotton swab in one-half dropperful Resinall K. Hold swab on the sore for 1 to 2 minutes. (Apply 3 to 4 times daily.)
- Nine Flavor Tea (3 tablets three times a day): Use for concurrent yin deficiency.

Corns and Calluses

Corns and calluses are caused by pressure and friction, producing a hardening and thickening of the skin. Shoes that do not fit well, and repetitive manual activities such as guitar playing or using a shovel may also cause corns and calluses. Medical attention is necessary if you are diabetic, or have a corn or callus that becomes ulcerated. Persistent corns or calluses on the feet can be removed by a podiatrist. To prevent corns on the feet wear comfortable shoes as much as possible or avoid wearing shoes.

Self Treatments

- Celandine (*Chelidonium majus*) herb: Apply the tincture topically to corns 2 times daily. Alternately, a soak for the feet or hands can be made by steeping 1 oz (28 grams) of dried celandine in 2 cups of boiling water for 20 to 30 minutes. If using fresh celandine, use 4 oz (112 grams) of fresh herb to 6 cups of boiling water. Soak the affected area twice daily for at least 10 minutes.
- White Flower Oil or wintergreen essential oil: Apply to corns and calluses to dissolve hardened skin and relieve pain (3 to 4 times daily).
- Fresh fig pulp remedy: Tape a piece of fresh fig pulp (or fresh pineapple) to the corn overnight. Remove in the morning and soak the foot in an Epsom salt bath. Gently rub the corn or callus with a pumice stone after soaking. Often the corn will dissolve within one week if this procedure is repeated each night. If fig or pineapple is unavailable, a salicylic acid pad (available at pharmacies) may be substituted.
- Carrot essential oil: Apply topically to dissolve corns and calluses (1 to 2 times daily).

Professional Treatments

- Resinall E (3 tablets three or four times a day): Take in addition to the above remedies.
- Resinall K: Apply topically (3 to 4 times daily). Use as a supplement to the above measures.

Dandruff

The shedding of dead skin from the scalp is a natural occurrence. Shedding of large flakes that are noticeable on hair or clothing is called dandruff. Dandruff is a mild form of seborrheic dermatitis—an itchy, scaly rash that occurs on the scalp, face, chest, and back (see section later in this chapter). Over-the-counter dandruff shampoos are usually helpful; however, they may contain allergens or other ingredients too harsh for some people. Gentler shampoos with natural ingredients are available at health food stores. One such product is Everclean Antidandruff Shampoo manufactured by Home Health.

To control dandruff, it is important to wash daily with a dandruff shampoo, leaving the lather on your head for several minutes. Rinse thoroughly and follow with an application of conditioner. Rinsing the hair with one-half cup of vinegar diluted in 1 quart of water may also help address the problem. If you have large flakes, along with scaling and itching around the nose, ears, or chest, you may have a more severe dermatitis, possibly eczema, for which a medical diagnosis should be made.

Self-Treatments

- Pyrithione zinc or selenium sulfide shampoos: Available over-the-counter (follow label directions).
- Pine tar shampoo: Available over-the-counter. Wash hair, letting the lather soak into the scalp. Then cover head with a shower cap for an hour or so. Use once daily until the dandruff clears.
- For even stronger results, mix the following essential oils with 2 oz of pure jojoba oil after shampooing: cedarwood (3 drops), cypress (5 drops), and juniper (5 drops). Massage a few tea-

spoons of this mixture into the scalp and let sit for 5 to 15 minutes.

- Vitamin A (20,000 to 50,000 IU daily). Vitamin A should be used cautiously during pregnancy; consult your health-care professional about dosages over 5,000 IU.
- Vitamin B complex (50 mg daily) plus PABA (100 mg daily): Used together for their synergistic effect.
- Broad-spectrum antioxidant (follow label directions).
- Black currant oil (at least 3,000 mg daily).

Professional Treatment

- Tinea therapy may be a useful part of dandruff treatment (see "Tinea" later in the chapter).

Dermatomyositis and Polymyositis

Dermatomyositis is a connective tissue disease characterized by muscle weakness, rash on the face, knuckles, elbows, knees, and ankles. There may also be pain, swelling, heat, and redness of the small joints. Diagnosis is confirmed through blood tests, electromyography (measurement of the electrical patterns of the muscles), and biopsy. This disease often affects women between 40 and 60 years old, and children between the ages of 5 and 15. Dermatomyositis may disappear within a few months; however, it can be fatal if the muscles of the tongue are affected or swallowing becomes difficult. Polymyositis shares the characteristic symptoms of dermatomyositis, but with polymyositis there is no skin rash.

Conventional treatment commonly involves rest and corticosteroids for the acute phase. As the condition improves, the corticosteroids are slowly reduced, and an exercise program is started when the condition has stabilized. Patients should be monitored for cancer, as dermatomyositis is sometimes associated with malignant tumors. Traditional Chinese medicine treatments for dermatomyositis vary depending on whether the patient exhibits symptoms of heat-toxin, cold-dampness, or deficiency.

Professional Treatments

- ◆ Mobility Three (3 tablets three times a day): Use for a cold-damp presentation. Signs and symptoms include muscle weakness, coldness of the hands, feet, and lower back, along with pain that worsens in cold-damp weather. The pulse is usually slow.
  - ▪ For extreme fatigue, cold muscles and joints, and a weak kidney pulse, Backbone (2 tablets four times a day) can be combined with Mobility Three (2 tablets four times a day).
- ◆ Marrow Plus (3 tablets three times a day): Use for signs of blood deficiency (pallor, weakness, or anemia) to nourish blood.
- ◆ Clear Heat (2 tablets four times a day) and Coptis Purge Fire (2 tablets four times a day): Use for a presentation that includes pain and weakness of the muscles and joints, high fever, and a dry throat.
  - ▪ As the heat symptoms recede use Clear Heat (2 tablets four times a day) and Mobility 2 (2 tablets four times a day).
- ◆ Loranthus (*sang ji sheng*) and carthamus (*hong hua*) wash: Use to promote blood circulation and reduce pain. Add 1 tsp each of loranthus and carthamus to 8 oz water. Simmer for 5 minutes, then steep for 15 minutes. Apply as a wash to the affected area 2 to 3 times daily.

- Clear Heat wash: Crush 6 tablets of Clear Heat and boil in 32 oz water for five minutes. Steep for another 10 minutes. Apply 2 to 3 times daily.
- Golden Yellow Ointment: Apply topically (1 to 3 times daily).

Diaper Rash

Diaper rash is irritation of the skin usually caused by contact with feces and urine. However, it may also be a sensitivity reaction to soaps, disposable diapers, and plastic pants. Typically the skin is red and irritated, although there may also be swollen areas and ulceration. Fungal diaper rash due to candida, is usually diagnosed by a doctor or nurse, and is characterized by smooth shiny skin, and a bright red rash with well-defined borders.

Diaper rash can be prevented by exposing the skin to air and sunlight. Preventive measures include abstaining from diaper use when possible, using cloth diapers that are loose fitting, and cleaning the area gently but thoroughly with each diaper change. After cleansing the area, rinse with a solution of one-eighth to 1 tbsp of baking soda mixed with 2 to 4 oz of water.

The standard biomedical approach is to use topical antifungal medication for diaper rash caused by candida. In addition, drying ointments are used to protect the skin from feces and urine. Hydrocortisone may be prescribed for a persistent diaper rash, but should not be used for more than 3 weeks or thinning of the skin may develop.

Self-Treatments

- Calendula ointment or lotion: Use to help reduce redness (1 to 2 times daily).

- Vitamin E topically (2 to 3 times daily). Break open 1 to 2 capsules and apply to the affected area.
- Skin clay: Use to help relieve oozing. Skin clay is available at health food stores. Dust clay on affected area after each diaper change.
- Acidophilus/bifidus: Children's PB8 (follow label directions).

Professional Treatments

- Oregano essential oil topically (2 to 3 times daily): Mix 1 part oregano essential oil with 1 to 2 parts vegetable oil.
- Biocidin compress: Mix 5 drops with 8 oz water, and apply as a compress (2 to 3 times daily).
- Vagistatin paste: Especially effective for fungal diaper rash. Add contents of one-half to 1 capsule to a small amount of water, apply to rash (1 to 3 times daily).

Drug Reaction Rash

Skin rashes that occur as a reaction to pharmaceutical medications, or even some herbs or nutritional supplements, are not uncommon. They may develop soon after taking the medication, herb, or supplement, or when a certain level of the medication, herb, or supplement has accumulated in the body. Common signs of drug rash are redness, itching, blistering and bleeding, or hives. A more severe reaction may involve nausea, vomiting, diarrhea, fever, seizures, irregular heartbeat, difficulty breathing, asthma, and increased or decreased urine flow.

If you have a skin rash that you believe is related to a medication, herb, or supplement, ask your healthcare professional about alternate products for your condition. Conventional treatment often uses antihistamines or cortisone cream to treat the rash.

Self-Treatments

- Take an oatmeal bath (see end of Chapter Two). Alternatively, use oatmeal soap until the rash is resolved. Oatmeal products may be contraindicated for persons sensitive to gluten.
- Bromelain enzyme formula (1,000 to 2,000 mg daily): Use to help reduce sensitivity.
- Antioxidant formula, such as Quercenol (2 tablets two times a day): Use to help reduce sensitivity over time.

Professional Treatments

- Xanthium Relieve Surface (3 tablets four to six times daily). To help increase the effectiveness of Xanthium Relieve Surface, add Coptis Purge Fire (2 to 3 tablets four times a day). Reduce dosage (to 1 tablet four times a day of each formula) if loose stools are noticed.
- Astra C (1 tablet three times a day) and/or Colostroplex (1 to 4 tablets daily): Use over 3 to 6 months to reduce hypersensitivity to the offending agent.

Dry Skin

The excretion of oils that lubricate our skin peaks in our teen years, then declines as we age. Dry skin is therefore a common phenomenon during the aging process. Dry skin is also more common in dry climates and during seasons when there is less moisture in the air. Antibacterial soap and excessive bathing or showering can also dry out the skin, causing the top layer of skin to become stiff and cracked. Once in this condition the skin can become red, irritated, and itchy.

To prevent dry skin, use oatmeal soaps and, if possible, try bathing less frequently. Spot-clean areas such as the underarms as needed. For severe problems during dry weather consider purchasing a humidifier for your home. Moisturizers that contain alpha-hydroxy acid help remove dead skin and are thus highly recommended. Increasing water intake can also help prevent skin dryness.

Self-Treatments

- ◆ Almond oil is a good moisturizer. To 30 ml of almond oil add 4 drops of lavender essential oil, 4 drops of geranium essential oil, and 1 drop of sandalwood essential oil. Apply 2 to 3 times daily.
- ◆ Flaxseeds: Include in diet. Grind 1 to 3 tablespoons whole flaxseeds daily. Mix the ground flaxseeds with one-half cup of juice and let the mixture congeal into a gelatin, or add to oatmeal or porridge.
- ◆ Fish oil (3 to 10 grams daily): Supplement with fish oil that contains EPA and DHA.
- ◆ Black currant oil (up to 3,000 mg daily).
- ◆ Vitamin E topically: Apply to troublesome spots and take internally (400 IU daily). Or break open capsules of vitamin E or antioxidant capsules and mix their contents into your moisturizing cream or sunscreen.
- ◆ Flax oil or walnut oil (1 to 2 tbsp daily): Use as a salad dressing.

Professional Treatments

♦ Nine Flavor Tea (3 tablets three times a day): Use for yin deficiency, characterized by heat in the palms or soles of feet, and thirst.

♦ Marrow Plus (3 tablets three times a day): Use for blood deficiency, characterized by pallor, anemia, fatigue, scanty periods in women.

♦ Spring Wind Ointment: Use for dry, itchy skin (3 to 4 times daily).

Case Study

Ann, a fifty-four-year-old administrator, complained of dry skin, low energy, and depression. She had previously undergone two major operations: a hysterectomy and removal of her gallbladder. Her thyroid was functioning normally according to biomedical tests, so hypothyroidism was ruled out as a source of her fatigue. Traditional Chinese medicine diagnosis revealed that her pulse was sinking and slow, and her tongue was pale.

We recommended the formula Shen Gem (2 tablets four times a day) to tonify the blood and thereby increase energy and nourish the skin. We also suggested almond oil topically for dryness. After two weeks, Ann noticed slight improvements in her energy and skin. Her tongue was less pale, but her pulse was unchanged. Ann continued the protocol for six months and experienced improvement in all symptoms.

Discussion: Surgical operations can be injurious to the blood and qi. According to Chinese medicine, dryness and itching of the skin is often due to a deficiency of blood. In Ann's case this was manifested by her pulse and tongue presentations.

Eczema (Dermatitis)

(See also Skin Allergies)

Dermatitis, literally, means "inflammation of the skin." Eczema is the overall term for any type of dermatitis, of which there are several: contact dermatitis, photodermatitis, atopic dermatitis, seborrheic dermatitis, and neurodermatitis, among others. Contact dermatitis occurs when the skin comes into contact with an irritant—either a substance that causes direct toxicity to the skin, or one that produces an allergic response. The allergic response may be immediate, or may take days to years to appear. Common irritants implicated in contact dermatitis include chemicals in personal grooming products such as soaps, lotions, perfumes, cosmetics, and contact lens cleaners. Ingredients in medications, chemicals found in household and industrial products such as cleaning agents are also known to cause reactions. In addition, certain plants, rubber, latex, and natural and synthetic fibers can be culprits. Contact dermatitis may show as redness, itching, blisters, or weepy sores. One common example of contact dermatitis is the reaction caused by poison oak, ivy, or sumac.

Photoallergic and phototoxic contact dermatitis are reactions that occur only after a topically applied substance is exposed to light. Commonly implicated substances in these light-dependent forms of contact dermatitis are aftershave lotions, sunscreens, and some perfumes.

Atopic dermatitis is the more severe and chronic kind of dermatitis that is often difficult to manage. This is the type of dermatitis that is popularly referred to as "eczema." Many individuals also have hay fever and asthma, which are also categorized as "atopic conditions." Thus, along with atopic dermatitis, these three conditions are known biomedically as the "atopic triad." Itching is a major problem in atopic dermatitis, as scratching the

100

lesions contributes to further development of the rash and more itching. Redness and scaling is often found in the creases of the elbows and knees, as well as on the eyelids, wrists, and neck. A family history of these problems is often present. Many individuals can indicate certain triggers, which range from dry skin to irritants and allergens to emotional stress, among others factors. Food additives appear to be culprits as well.[15]

The symptoms of seborrheic dermatitis are redness, itching, and scaling on the face, behind the ears, or over the breastbone. Stubborn, itchy dandruff that may be greasy and reddened is often considered a type of seborrheic dermatitis. With neurodermatitis, nervous tension and anxiety lead to itching and scratching. Stasis dermatitis is thickening and itching of the skin around the ankles where the skin may be inflamed and ulcers may form.

For contact and atopic dermatitis, the first step in treatment (and in preventing future outbreaks) is to avoid the offending trigger(s). Standard biomedical treatment for dermatitis includes applying corticosteroid creams and use of oral antihistamines. But such treatment, while helpful for acute itching, is slowly losing favor because it is not effective for long-term management. In addition, there are the well-known side effects of prolonged use of steroids. Other treatments such as the use of ultraviolet or sunlamps are sometimes helpful. Newer agents such as immunemodulators are currently being studied. With atopic dermatitis, meticulous self-management is crucial in keeping the condition under control. In addition to identifying trigger(s), measures such as wearing loose, non-wool clothing to prevent itching, keeping the skin clean through bathing, and applying moisturizer immediately after bathing to avoid dry skin, are important elements of self-management.

In cases of dermatitis that are stress-related, such as neurodermatitis, stress reduction techniques may be helpful. To prevent persistent scratching, dressings that are difficult to remove (thus prohibiting scratching) may be used. In extreme cases, physicians may administer sedative drugs. For more information, see the Skin Allergy section.

Self-Treatments

- The "Digestive Clearing Program" may help alleviate and prevent dermatitis. (See Appendix.)
- Identify food sensitivities and allergens and eliminate them from your diet. Many persons improve after eliminating dairy products and/or gluten-containing foods such as wheat, oat, barley, and rye. Shellfish is an allergen frequently implicated in eczema. Individuals who have eczema as well as digestive problems may also want to eliminate beans, especially soybeans, for two to six weeks. (See "Food Sensitivity.")
- Increase essential fatty acids by eating fatty fish such as salmon, mackerel, anchovies, and herring; or use fish oil supplements containing anti-inflammatory properties such as EPA, DHA, or cod liver oil (3 to 4 g daily for one month, then reduced to 1 to 2 g daily). Flax oil and black current oil are good substitutes. Flax oil can be used in salad dressing (1 tsp three times a day).
- Zinc (15 to 60 mg daily).
- Vitamin A (10,000 to 50,000 IU daily). Vitamin A should be used cautiously during pregnancy; consult your health-care professional about dosages over 5,000 IU.
- Bioflavonoids (1,000 to 2,000 mg daily).
- Use mild oatmeal or glycerine soap for bathing. Pat dry and apply moisturizing lotion.
- Dead sea salts placed in bath (follow label directions).
- Essential oils:
  - For bath use every 2 to 3 days: Add 4 drops geranium, 4 drops lavender, and 2 drops juniper to warm bath water.

- For topical use: Mix 5 drops lavender, 5 drops German chamomile, 5 drops tagetes, and 5 drops yarrow in 2 tbsp vegetable oil and 40 drops jojoba oil. Apply 2 to 3 times daily.
- Comfrey wash: Add 1 tsp to 8 oz boiling water, cover and steep for 15 minutes. Apply 1 to 2 times daily. Avoid using on open lesions.
- Use stress reduction techniques such as meditation, prayer, yoga, or qigong.

Professional Treatments

- Xanthium Relieve Surface (3 tablets 4 to 6 times daily): Use for contact dermatitis.
- Skin Balance with Six Gentlemen (2 to 3 tablets, 3 to 4 times daily, each formula): Use for any type of dermatitis accompanied by cold signs such as indigestion, bloating, and loose stools.
- Skin Balance with Coptis Purge Fire (2 to 3 tablets of each formula three to four times a day): Use for any type of dermatitis accompanied by heat signs such as extremely red skin, thirst, and constipation.
- Skin Balance with Marrow Plus (2 to 3 tablets of each formula three to four times a day): Use for any type of dermatitis, except contact dermatitis accompanied by blood deficiency.
- Resinall K topically (3 times daily): Use for itching and cracked skin. It may be combined with vegetable oil as desired.
- Spring Wind Ointment (3 times daily): Use for dry itching.
- Dictamus 13 (3 tablets three to four times per day): Use for itching without heat signs.
- High-quality probiotics, such as Lactobacillus GG (1 capsule daily, on an empty stomach): Use for any type of dermatitis.

- Whole dandelion plants: For any type of dermatitis, add a handful to 1 quart of water and simmer for 20 minutes. Drink 1 to 3 cups daily. Reduce if loose stools occur.
- Mango skin: For any type of dermatitis. Put skin in a pot, pour water to just cover the mango skin. Simmer 20 to 30 minutes. Let cool, and wash the affected area 3 times daily.
- Coconut oil: Use for neurodermatitis. Apply topically 2 to 3 times daily.

Case Studies

Case #1

Inga, a twenty-three-year-old model, had suffered from eczema (atopic dermatitis) ever since moving to the United States from Sweden two years earlier. Her chief complaint was dry skin affecting the entire body. In addition, she had irritable bowel syndrome, headaches, and anxiety. The cortisone creams she had been prescribed provided only temporary relief. She had also tried homeopathy and acupuncture but with minimal improvement. Traditional Chinese medicine diagnosis revealed that her pulse was wiry, and her tongue slightly purple.

We suggested she keep a food diary over the next week. In the meantime, we recommended that she take Skin Balance (2 tablets three times a day) and use a topical zinc preparation to be applied twice daily. One week later, she reported modest improvements: there was less itching and dryness; however, the skin on her elbows and hands was still thick and cracked. Her pulse and tongue were unchanged. Upon reviewing her food journal, we noticed a propensity of gluten-containing foods such as breads and oats, and recommended she try a gluten-free diet. We further suggested she take black currant capsules (6 per day) and add flax or hemp oil to her daily salads. She continued with the internal herbs and topical zinc preparation.

Inga followed this protocol for another month and experienced great improvement. She noticed that her skin itched after eating bread, so she eliminated bread and oats from her diet completely. With this change, all itching stopped. In addition to these improvements, her elbows and hands were smoother and less red. She remained on this protocol for several months with complete resolution of the dermatitis.

Case #2

Jonathan, a five-year-old, had very itchy, red eczema (atopic dermatitis) all over his body. He had the condition since he was one. His mother indicated that the eczema was probably from food allergy. Traditional Chinese medicine diagnosis revealed that Jonathan's pulse was rapid, and his tongue had a gray-yellow coating.

We recommended to his mother that all dairy products be eliminated from Jonathan's diet for a two-week trial period. We also suggested that he take the formula Skin Balance (1 to 2 tablets two times a day) and a fish oil preparation rich in EPA and DHA (one-third the adult dose). Within two weeks, Jonathan's eczema was fifty percent better. His mother was so pleased with this result that she decided to keep him on a dairy-free diet. After four weeks the eczema had improved by ninety percent.

Case #3

Tracie, a twenty-four-year-old administrative assistant, had severe eczema (atopic dermatitis) for ten years. Her skin was pale but very itchy and there were lesions on her hands, fingers, and elbows. The eczema was exacerbated by stress, and by sugar, processed foods, and fats, and especially by rich and creamy foods. She had been prescribed topical and oral corticosteroids, which suppressed the symptoms as long as she used them continually. However, the symptoms recurred whenever she discontinued the medications. In addition, she had long-standing digestive problems such as intestinal bloating, gas, and abdominal cramping. She also had a history of anemia and infrequent menstrual periods. At times, several months would pass with no menses. When she did have a period, it was accompanied by severe cramps and discomfort. Traditional Chinese medicine diagnosis found that her pulse was slow and wiry, and her tongue was dry and purple with red dots.

We recommended she apply a topical zinc spray to her skin (3 times daily) followed by Spring Wind ointment (3 times daily). We also suggested Skin Balance (2 tablets two times a day) and urged her to keep a food journal that we could review during her next appointment.

Two weeks later she complained of loose stools and increased bloating, but also noted that the itching had improved. Her pulse was weak and slow, and her tongue was red. Upon reviewing her food journal, we noted that she had eaten large amounts of soy and gluten-containing foods such as bread and oats. We therefore suggested a two-week trial eliminating such foods. As Tracie was a vegetarian and already underweight, she was concerned about getting adequate protein, so we recommended rice protein powders.

We also suggested she discontinue Skin Balance as it may have been too strongly detoxifying, thereby creating more gastrointestinal upset. Instead, we decided to approach her skin condition from the "inside out" by using internal herbs to resolve her digestive tract imbalances. In Chinese medicine, the large intestine is paired with the lung. The lung, in turn, is associated with the skin. Since she had signs of coldness (bloating, irregular periods), we recommended that she take Six Gentlemen (3 tablets three times a day) with fennel tea (1 to 2 cups, 3 times per day) to warm up her system.

Two weeks later, Tracie's digestion had improved and she experienced less itching. Although the lesions remained, they were less red and purple. Her pulse was slow and weak in the lung position, but her tongue was normal. She continued the protocol with the addition of Eight Treasures (1 tablet three times a day) to nourish her blood. We suggested this low dosage to prevent the cloying nature of the blood tonic from exacerbating her digestive symptoms.

Three weeks later the eczema on Tracie's hands and fingers was worse. She reported having one stressful week at work and the reintroduction of wheat to her diet, which she noticed made her skin worse. We suggested she add pearl barley to her diet to benefit the skin. She was also asked to make a wash with licorice root in order to soothe her hands and fingers, and follow it with zinc spray and Spring Wind ointment. We also recommended she increase her intake of fatty acids with black currant capsules (500 mg, 6 per day with meals) and by using flax oil as part of her salad dressing. She continued with Six Gentlemen (3 tablets three times a day) and Eight Treasures (1 tablet three times a day). We worked with Tracie for over six months, occasionally adding in Skin Balance (1 tablet three times a day) and Dictamus 13 (3 tablets three times a day) to help improve her skin. After six months her skin had cleared, and remained so one year later.

Case #4

Richard, a thirty-four-year-old consultant, complained of eczema (atopic dermatitis) and constant itching, which he had for the past fourteen years. In addition to eczema he reported allergies to dust, smoke, feathers, pollen, dogs, and cats. He also had constipation, and said that he never sweated, even during exercise. Traditional Chinese medicine diagnosis revealed that his pulse was thin, rapid, and slightly irregular, and his tongue was red. His face had a black-purple tinge, indicating kidney weakness and blood stagnation. He appeared exhausted.

We counseled him to drink at least 64 oz of water per day, to which he replied that he had been told by a Chinese herbalist to drink only four glasses of tea per day. We advised him that tea actually contributes to dehydration and urged him to drink more fluids other than tea. We also recommended topical Spring Wind Ointment as well as flax oil (1 to 2 tbsp daily), and fish oil (4 g daily). We also asked him to take the remedies Skin Balance (3 tablets three times a day) and Gentle Senna (1 to 2 tablets three times a day).

Richard had already achieved some results with Dead Sea bath salts, so we encouraged him to continue. We treated Richard for over six months. After two months the Gentle Senna was stopped and Eight Treasures begun (3 tablets three times a day). Skin Balance was continued at the same dosage. He continued on these formulas for the next four months, at the end of which his eczema improved by eighty percent.

Case #5

Joy, an eleven-year-old girl, had eczema (atopic dermatitis) with dry, itchy skin affecting the whole body, especially the elbows. Traditional Chinese medicine diagnosis revealed her pulse was rapid, and her tongue reddish purple.

We advised Joy's mother to try eliminating dairy products and gluten-containing foods from Joy's diet for a six-week trial period and, either concurrently or subsequently, to eliminate corn, shellfish, chocolate, tomatoes, nuts, and beans. We also recommended Skin Balance (1 tablet three times a day) to clear the skin and Marrow Plus (2 tablets three times a day) to nourish blood.

We saw Joy two weeks later and there was a slight improvement; however, her skin was still very dry and itchy, and her pulse and tongue were unchanged. We recommended Resinall K topically twice a day, in addition to the herbs. As it was hard for Joy to eliminate cow's milk, we suggested to her mother that she gradually incorporate rice or soymilk into Joy's diet. We also advised that she take a multimineral formula to ensure that her calcium intake was adequate. It was also challenging for the mother to prepare gluten-free meals, so we guided her toward alternatives.

After four weeks Joy's skin had improved greatly. The mother reported that the itching had subsided by about fifty percent. As Joy's one elbow still had lesions, we recommended cleaning the area with soapy water then applying Resinall K topically (2 times daily). For the next three months Joy continued using the herbal supplements and Resinall K. Now her dermatitis flares up only occasionally during times of stress.

Case #6

Jeremy, a fifty-year-old contractor, complained of itching due to eczema (atopic dermatitis) over his entire body. Additionally, he had insomnia. Traditional Chinese medicine diagnosis revealed that his pulse was wiry and his tongue was red.

We suggested he eliminate alcohol, sweets, fruit, and wheat from his diet for a trial period of two weeks. We also recommended the herbal formulas Phellostatin (1 tablet three times a day the first week, 2 to 3 tablets three times a day thereafter) and Skin Balance (1 tablet three times a day the first week, 2 tablets three times a day thereafter).

After two weeks Jeremy reported a fifty percent improvement in the itching, but no change in the insomnia. His pulse was less wiry, but his tongue was still red. We advised that he continue with the herbs as directed and that twice a day he apply a mixture of lavender essential oil (2 drops) to safflower oil (2 tsp). We also suggested that he wash with oatmeal soap or aloe soap, rather than standard commercial brands.

After one month Jeremy reported an eighty to ninety percent reduction in the itching as long as he followed the diet and took the recommended herbs. As of this writing, he continues to follow this protocol.

Case #7

Brendon, an energetic two-year-old, was covered, head to toe, with red, itchy eczema (atopic dermatitis). He also had scaling of the skin behind the knees, and postnasal drip with clear discharge.

We recommended to his mother that he be put on a dairy-free diet. We also suggested children's PB-8 acidophilus (1 tsp daily) and Six Gentlemen (1 tablet two times a day, ground up and added to hot water, cooled, and put into apple or grape juice). Acidophilus and/or bifidus products are common holistic remedies for pediatric eczema. Six Gentlemen was used to improve digestive function and gently resolve phlegm.

After one month and only slight improvement we began suspecting other potential allergens, such as citrus, egg, wheat, shellfish, and chocolate, so we recommended eliminating these foods from Brendon's diet. At this point we also recommended cool compresses with chamomile essential oil. We also suggested black currant oil (contents of 2 capsules squeezed and added to the PB-8 acidophilus) and Skin Balance (1 tablet per day) in addition to the Six Gentlemen. After another month, Brendon's condition improved substantially. Brendon remains on the protocol, and will stop the Skin Balance when his skin no longer has a red tinge.

Frostbite and Chilblains (Pernio)

Frostbite is cold and numbness caused by exposure to temperatures below freezing. Upon warming, the frostbitten area becomes red, swollen, and painful. If you suspect someone has suffered frostbite, warm the body and affected area as rapidly as possible by either submerging in, or using a wet cloth soaked in warm water (between 104°F and 107°F, or 40°C to 42°C) for twenty-minute periods. You may need to begin with cooler temperatures and warm the water up gradually from lukewarm to hot. Severe cases of frostbite may lead to ulceration and even gangrene, so it is imperative in such cases to seek medical attention immediately. Vasodilating drugs, or anticoagulants such as ibuprofen may be prescribed. Chilblains, or pernio, refer to long-lasting or recurrent inflammation, itching, and swelling after exposure to mild cold or damp cold.

In China, acupuncture is often used to speed healing after the acute stage of frostbite. Standard acupuncture, plum-blossom needling causing a small amount of bleeding, as well as moxibustion, all stimulate circulation, thus promoting recovery of the skin and tissues.

Self-Treatments

- Ginger powder tea: Steep one-third to one-half tsp in 8 oz of hot water. Take 3 times daily for a few days until feeling returns to the affected area.
- Ginger powder soak: Boil 1 tsp ginger powder per 8 oz water for 5 minutes. Let cool, then soak the affected area 3 times daily for a few days until feeling returns to the affected area.
- Red Tiger Balm: Use topically to restore sensation. Apply topically 3 times daily.

111

Professional Treatments

- ◆ Channel Flow and Flavonex (2 tablets four times a day for each formula): Use to help promote circulation. Take until feeling is restored to the affected area.

Genital Herpes

Genital herpes is transmitted by sexual contact. Blisters or ulcers may form in the genital area, anus, buttocks, and thighs. Invisible sores may form inside the cervix or urethra. The sores typically begin as small red bumps that become water blisters that ooze or bleed. It is important to see a physician as early as possible to get a thorough diagnosis, and to see if you have an additional sexually transmitted disease. Acyclovir, an antiviral drug, may be prescribed. It is important to keep the sores clean and dry and to abstain from sex while the sores are present. Itching or burning can precede the actual outbreak; this is known as the prodromal stage. Taking herbs at this stage in many cases enables you from getting a full-blown infection. Emphasize high lysine foods: fish, turkey, chicken, beef, dairy, beans, eggs, sprouts, nutritional yeast, vegetables; avoid or minimize arginine-containing foods: nuts, seeds, brown rice, oats, raisins, caffeine, coconut, carob, eggplant, green peppers, tomatoes, mushrooms, garbanzo beans, sugar; chocolate, and alcohol.

Stress reduction is very important for preventing and lessening outbreaks. For women, hormone-regulating herbs can also be helpful at treating the herpes outbreaks that regularly occur before, during, or after menstruation.

Self-Treatments

◆ Lemon Balm tea as a wash. Steep 1 tbsp of lemon balm in 8 oz of water; cover for 15 minutes and apply topically 3 times a day.

◆ Zinc/antioxidants to prevent outbreaks. Use as directed.

◆ St. John's Wort salve/oil applied topically three times a day.

◆ Licorice as a wash. Simmer 1 tsp of licorice root for 10 minutes. Steep 10 minutes longer and apply topically with a handcloth or cottonball.

◆ Echinacea and goldenseal products can speed the healing process. Use at least 2,000 mg daily.

Professional Treatments

◆ Coptis Purge Fire: For acute outbreak, take 3 tablets 4 to 6 times per day; reduce if loose stools are noticed.

◆ Astra Isatis: For prevention, take 2 to 3 tablets three times a day. At the prodromal stage take 9 tablets in order to prevent the outbreak.

◆ Resinall K: May be applied topically to lesions to reduce pain, 1 to 3 times daily. Clean area well first.

Case Study

Bob is a thirty-six-year-old cab driver with genital herpes. In the month before he consulted us, he had stopped taking acyclovir, and had suffered a major outbreak. When he came to the clinic he was in the prodromal stage of another outbreak. His pulse was rapid and his tongue red. We recommended he take nine tablets of Astra Isatis, and advised him to take another nine tablets as soon as he got home. We instructed him to take another dosage at night if he still felt like he was going to have an outbreak. We suggested he reduce or eliminate sweets, especially chocolate, alcohol, nuts, and that he increase his intake of vegetables.

Bob called up the next day saying that he thought the herbs had knocked out the outbreak. We suggested he continue taking Astra Isatis at a lower dosage (3 tablets three times a day). Bob continued to take Astra Isatis over the next year. He stopped once during this period, and got an outbreak, for which Coptis Purge Fire (3 tablets, 4 to 6 per day) was recommended, along with lemon balm compresses.

Discussion: It is interesting to note that when Bob got the outbreak, he had been under a lot of stress caring for his mother who was hospitalized, and as a result was drinking alcohol every night and was unable to eat a good diet. Chocolate and nuts contain arginine, which is thought to stimulate herpes replication. Alcohol is warming in nature.

Genital Warts

Genital warts (codylomata acuminata) are highly contagious. Small growths in the genital area are commonly found on the penis, between the genitals and anus, around the anus, around the vagina, or in the cervix. Genital warts are spread by sexual contact. It may take months or even a year after infection for a wart to appear.

Even after a wart has been removed, the virus can remain in the bodily tissue, leading to another outbreak. If you have a genital wart, see a physician or Planned Parenthood as soon as possible for treatment and to make sure you have not acquired any other sexually-transmitted diseases. As genital warts are associated with increased risk of cervical cancer, it is important for women diagnosed with genital warts to get a yearly PAP. Genital warts can be removed by freezing (cryosurgery) or laser. The sexual partner(s) of the infected should be examined.

Self-Treatments

- Vitamin A and antioxidants may help reduce latent virus.
- Power Mushrooms (3 tablets two times a day) to strengthen immunity.
- Astra 8 (3 tablets two times a day) to strengthen immunity.

Professional Treatments

- Vagistatin may be used to reduce virus (contents of 2 caps applied topically at night).
- Astra Isatis can be used to boost the immune system and reduce latent virus (3 tablets three times a day).
- Unlocking is typically combined with Astra Isatis if there is pain or heat signs. It can be used by itself short-term (2 tablets of each formula four times a day).

Case Studies

Case #1

Sylvie, a forty-six-year-old designer, complained of genital warts. She was a vegetarian and a great believer in natural therapies, so she wanted to try herbs before resorting to Western medicine. We replied that the best way to treat the warts was by freezing or laser surgery, but that the herbs could be taken to support her immune system and attack the virus, which remains latent even though warts are removed. We strongly recommended she have her partner see a medical doctor or Planned Parenthood to get treatment, and that he also take herbs. Sylvie's pulse was wiry and her tongue was red. We recommended Astra Isatis (3 tablets three times a day), which she continued to take for the next year. She stopped for a brief time when she caught a flu, and when she was on vacation.

Case #2

Lisa is a twenty-three-year-old massage practitioner with genital warts. Her pulse was thin and wiry and her tongue was reddish purple. She was referred to a physician for cryosurgery (freezing the warts), and was advised to take Astra Isatis (3 tablets three times a day), which has immune tonifying and antiviral properties, according to Chinese research. She returned four weeks after the surgery. She said she felt cold in the uterus since the surgery, and tired. She blamed herself for having unprotected sex, which is how we believe she acquired the warts. Her pulse was unchanged and her tongue was pale with a purple tinge. Therefore, we recommended Astra Isatis (2 tablets four times a day) and Eight Treasures (2 tablet four times a day) to build blood.

One month later she returned feeling much better. Her pulse was wiry but her tongue was normal. We recommended she continue to take Astra Isatis (2 tablets two times a day) for at least three months to help rid the body of latent virus.

Hair Loss

Hair loss can be due to age, hormonal changes, infections, skin disease, reactions to drugs (especially chemotherapy), malnutrition, cancer, radiation, and poisoning. Male pattern baldness (androgenic alopecia) is an inherited condition that depends upon age and hormones. Cosmetic solutions include topical minoxidil (Rogaine), which only helps some of those who use it, wigs, hair transplants, or surgery. Propecia or hormone therapy may be recommended in some cases.

Loss of hair at the crown or at the hairline and general thinning of hair characterize female pattern baldness. It is normal for hair to thin as we age; however, significant hair loss is typically the result of having inherited genes that tend toward baldness. Hair loss may also be caused by hormonal changes such as those during menopause, hair disorders, pregnancy, poor nutrition, and medical treatments such as chemotherapy and radiotherapy. Alopecia areata is a common condition, where circular bald patches develop suddenly. The cause of alopecia areata is suspected to be stress, genetic predisposition, and an autoimmune reaction to one's hair follicles. In ninety percent of the cases, the hair grows back within two years. It makes sense to see a physician to get a diagnosis after any sudden hair loss.

Self-Treatments

In a double-blind study with alopecia areata, 44 percent of those who rubbed essential oils into their scalps showed improvement in bald patches. Combine 2 drops thyme, 3 drops of lavender, 3 drops of rosemary, 2 drops of cedarwood with 4 tsp of carrier oil and one-half tsp jojoba.[16]

- ◆ Horsetail tea: Boil 1 tsp of powdered herb in water and let it steep for 10 minutes. Strain. Drink 3 cups per day. Horsetail is rich in the mineral silica.

- Standing on your head for 20 to 40 breaths will help bring circulation to your scalp. Consult a yoga practitioner to do this properly.

Professional Treatments

- Astra Essence contains the herb he show wu (3 tablets two to three times a day for 6 to 12 months).
- Thymus preparations for immune conditions. Use topically as directed.
- Take up to 8,000 mcg of biotin, which is used to empirically treat scalp conditions.

Case Study

Brenda is a thirty-nine-year-old executive who was under a lot of work-related pressure and was going through a divorce. Her complaints were stress, hair loss, and indigestion. Her pulse was wiry, and her tongue was red-purple, and dry. We recommended she take Ease 2 along with Astra Essence, one tablet of each formula four times a day the first week, and two of each four times a day thereafter. Astra Essence was used to reduce hair loss and to build her kidney energy (hair depends upon the kidney in TCM) and Ease 2 is used for regulating liver qi stagnation. After three weeks, she reported she felt calmer, her digestion was better, and she felt that there was less hair in the shower after washing. Her pulse was less wiry and the tongue was unchanged. After several months she felt there had been a definite decrease in hair loss.

After four months of taking the herbs, she came down with a gastrointestinal infection and was prescribed antibiotics by her medical doctor. After a course of antibiotics she came back complaining that the Astra Essence had stopped working after taking the antibiotics. She also complained of anger and palpitations. Her pulse was wiry, and her tongue was red and dry. At this point, we suggested she have her heartbeat monitored by a medical doctor. We also suggested Ease 2 and Calm Spirit, 2 tablets of each formula four times a day, in order to stabilize the emotions. We also recommended that she see a colleague who is an acupuncturist; however, she said she was afraid of needles. We urged her to resume the stress reduction program she had started, but was not consistent in following.

After three weeks, she felt the herbs had helped her feel more peaceful. At this point, her pulse was calmer, though her tongue was unchanged. We suggested she resume taking Ease 2 and Astra Essence (2 tablets of each formula four times a day). Within two weeks, she remarked that she thought the herbs were once again reducing the hair loss, as evidenced by the reduced amount of hair in the shower.

Hives (Urticaria)

Hives are itchy, red welts appearing on the surface of the skin. Angioedema is similar; however, the welts are larger and affect both the surface of the skin and subcutaneous structures. Onset is usually sudden. Both hives and angioedema are allergic reactions that may be caused by foods, medications, stress, insect bites, illness, cold, heat, light, pollen, and animal dander. Identifying and avoiding the offending agent is the best preventive measure. Conventional medical treatments include antihistamines, corticosteroids, epinephrine, and topical applications to stop itching. Foods often implicated in both of these conditions are preserved meats, fish and shellfish, nuts, eggs, milk, strawberries, and foods containing preservatives or artificial colors.

Self-Treatments

- A daily stress reduction protocol can be very helpful for people with chronic hives, since stress can heighten the body's sensitivity level.
- Vitamin C (1,000 to 10,000 mg daily): Use the buffered or mineral ascorbate kind and Quercetin (500 to 3,000 mg daily) to reduce allergic response.
- High-potency bromelain and companion enzymes such as papain (500 to 1,000 mg three times daily).
- Witch hazel: Use topically during the early stages of an outbreak to help alleviate discomfort.
- Digestive Harmony (2 to 3 tablets three times a day): Use during an outbreak. It tends to reduce the severity of allergic reactions.

Professional Treatments

- Xanthium Relieve Surface (3 tablets four times a day). To stop allergic reactions combine with Astra C (1 tablet four times a day) to help the immune system.
- Xanthium Relieve Surface (2 tablets four times a day) with either Coptis Purge Fire (3 tablets four times a day) or Clear Heat (2 tablets four times a day): Use for hives caused by infection (flu, hepatitis, infectious mononucleosis). Clear Heat can be used topically as a wash.
- Peppermint essential oil: Mix 5 drops with 1 tsp of vegetable oil or with 8 oz water, and apply as a cool compress 2 to 3

times daily. Or, apply oil directly to the weals and at acu-points LI 11 and SP 10 to help speed resolution of hives. Any of the following ear points may also be used: Shenmen, Adrenal Gland, Endocrine Point, Corresponding Body Area, Allergy Point, Antihistamine, Lung 1 and 2, Contralaeral Lung, and Ipsilateral Lung to promote resolation of the hives.

Case Studies

Case #1

Madeline, a twenty-year-old secretary, had hives which were unrelieved by standard biomedical treatment. The hives felt "itchy, tingly, and heavy." She also complained of dry skin, excessive sweating, hay fever, sinus pressure, reactive diarrhea after eating certain foods, and occasional constipation. All symptoms were worse in hot weather. Traditional Chinese medicine diagnosis revealed that her pulse was thin, deep, and weak. Her tongue was pale and dry.

We recommended Madeline give up cereal and dairy products for two weeks, as she noticed a tendency toward diarrhea after eating these foods. We inquired about sodas since she had arrived at the clinic with a diet soda in her hand. She reported drinking four to six per day. We urged her to stop drinking sodas as soon as possible because the chemicals in the ingredients were causing accumulation of heat in her system, and to drink 64 or more ounces of water per day instead. We also recommended that she increase her intake of fresh vegetables and fruits, and substitute lean meat for cheese as an alternate protein source. In terms of herbal formulas, we suggested Nine Flavor Tea (3 tablets three times a day) to nourish yin and Coptis Purge Fire (1 tablet three times a day) to rid her body of excess heat. Colostroplex

(1 or 2 tablets daily) was also given to help strengthen her stomach and intestines, remove toxins via the stools, and reduce food reactivity.

A week later, Madeline reported improvement in both the hives and diarrhea, though her skin still felt dry. Her pulse and tongue were unchanged. We recommended she increase the dosage of Coptis Purge Fire (to 3 tablets three times a day). She said she had reduced her soda intake to one per day but was having difficulty drinking so much water. We urged her to eliminate the soda completely and suggested keeping a water bottle with her to sip from throughout the day. We added that peppermint tea could be substituted for some of the water if it would help increase her fluid intake.

After another week she said she felt much better from the increased dose of herbs and was starting to feel like her old self. She had become constipated the previous week, so we suggested she reduce the Colostroplex (to 1 tablet per day or 1 every other day). Madeline came for appointments infrequently after that, mainly to get herbs when her symptoms recurred due to stress.

Case #2 Hives with Sjögren's Syndrome

Sandra, a seventy-three-year old, came to our clinic presenting with signs of angioedema. She also had Sjögren's syndrome. Her principle symptoms were recurrent hives, edema, and purpura, which were relieved by antihistamines. In addition, she had episodes of extreme fatigue, difficulty concentrating, gas and bloating, loose stools, joint pain, and generalized sensations of dryness and heat. Traditional Chinese medicine diagnosis revealed that her pulse was choppy and thin, and her tongue was red with red spots and had a yellow coating.

We recommended the formula Colostroplex (2 tablets two times a day) to improve the function of her digestive system and to bind and eliminate toxins. Sandra was also advised to take Quercenol (2 tablets two times a day), which is a broad-spectrum antioxidant, Nine Flavor Tea (2 tablets three times a day), and Lithospermum 15 (2 tablets three times a day). We suggested that she try a gluten-free diet, including at least one bowl of rice every day, and to eat organically raised meat or fresh fish, especially salmon. She was also asked to increase her intake of vegetables, to eliminate all dairy products from her diet, and to minimize sweets, processed, and greasy foods. After two weeks, Sandra reported fewer bouts of loose stools and an apparent reduction in hives. Her pulse and tongue were unchanged, though. We then recommended increasing the Nine Flavor Tea and Lithospermum 15 (to 2 tablets each three times a day) while continuing with the other herbs and supplements.

After following this protocol for four weeks, Sandra reported increased gas and bloating, but less hives. Her pulse was slightly less choppy, and her tongue coating was less yellow and thick. At this point, we recommended that she temporarily discontinue Nine Flavor Tea, as the yin tonifying herbs it contains may be difficult to digest. The formula Calm Spirit (2 tablets three times a day) was substituted instead. Calm Spirit contains yin tonics that are more readily digestible as well as enzymes that function as antioxidants.

After one month, Sandra reported a slight improvement in her energy, considerably reduced sensations of heat and dryness, and a dramatic reduction in hives. Her pulse was thin and irregular, and her tongue was red and dry. We then recommended Astra Essence (3 tablets three times a day) and Calm Spirit (3 tablets three times a day) along with the Quercenol (2 tablets two times a day) and reduce the Colostroplex (to 1 tablet two times a day).

Sandra remained on this protocol for several months. The result was a significant increase in energy, a reduction in joint pain, fewer sensations of dryness and heat, and far fewer out-breaks of hives and edema. The outbreaks she did have could usually be traced to consumption of dairy products, wheat, and certain fruits.

Discussion: Sandra's was a case of yin deficiency. The yin deficiency manifested as constant sensations of dryness and heat. The formula Lithospermum 15 contains heat-clearing herbs, tonifying herbs, as well as those that promote blood circulation. Astra Essence strongly tonifies qi, blood, yin, and yang, and was given to address Sandra's signs of deficiency, fatigue, and poor concentration.

Nine Flavor Tea was recommended initially to strongly nourish yin; however, its cloying yin tonics may have been too difficult for her to digest. Substituting Calm Spirit seemed to achieve the goal of nourishing yin without these untoward effects. It also helped her feel calmer, which may have had a positive effect on her nervous system, thus resulting in fewer outbreaks of hives. Colostroplex was recommended to help heal her gastrointestinal system by binding toxins and eliminating them through the feces; it also specifically treats diarrhea and loose stools, and may reduce food sensitivities by enhancing gastrointestinal immunity if taken for three to six consecutive months.

Case #3 Mastocytosis

Carrie, a twenty-two-year-old student, had severe hives, abdominal pain, and diarrhea. She was diagnosed with mastocytosis, a condition also known as urticaria pigmentosa, which is characterized by itchy, irregular, yellow or orange-brown swellings. Her physician had prescribed prednisone (20 mg per day), Zantac, and antihistamines. Traditional Chinese medicine diagnosis revealed that her pulse was weak, and her tongue was purple with spots and had a gray coating in the rear.

We recommended she try an elimination diet for two weeks that focused on eating vegetables, lean protein, rice, and millet. We also suggested the formula Colostroplex (2 tablets three times a day) to stop diarrhea and improve her immune system, and Skin Balance (1 tablet three times a day). When she returned two weeks later, Carrie said she was under too much stress to try the elimination diet, and that although her diarrhea had lessened, some days there was as much, if not more, cramping. Her pulse was weak, and her tongue unchanged. We suggested she add Quiet Digestion to her protocol (2 tablets three times a day) and that she begin to eliminate gluten-containing foods as well as soy and dairy products.

After another two weeks, she looked more energetic. Both the hives and the diarrhea were much less severe, though she was still having abdominal pain. At this point, Carrie was asked to discontinue Skin Balance as it contains purgatives that can be difficult on the digestive system. The formula Clear Heat (2 tablets three times a day) was prescribed instead. The other herbs in the protocol remained the same.

Three weeks later when Carrie returned, she indicated that the hives were finally manageable and, with her doctor's permission, she reduced the prednisone and antihistamines. She attributed her improvements to the herbs and to eliminating milk and cheese from her diet.

Case #4

Neil, a fifty-year-old plumber, had recurring hives on his arms and legs for four years. He also complained of headaches, constipation, and frequent urination. Traditional Chinese medicine diagnosis revealed that his pulse was slippery, and his tongue was pale with a thick yellow coating in the rear. Neil admitted that his diet was poor and that he drank nightly.

Suspecting that Neil might have a fungal infection because his symptoms were worse in moldy environments, we suggested he first adopt an antifungal diet, eliminating alcohol, sweets, dairy, and wheat, and take Skin Balance (2 to 3 tablets three times a day). As his bowels were moving only once every three days, we also recommended that he eat 1 to 2 teaspoons a day of ground flaxseeds, use flax oil on salads, and increase his intake of water and vegetables.

After two weeks the hives had improved despite the fact that Neil had reduced, but not eliminated, alcohol and sweets. His pulse was unchanged and his tongue coating was less thick. As he was still constipated we suggested he increase his dosage of Skin Balance (to 4 tablets three times a day), as this formula contains herbs that promote intestinal health. After one month the hives were significantly better and Neil was experiencing headaches only on the weekends, which we were able to correlate to weekend drinking. Neil stayed on the protocol for six months. During this time Ecliptex (2 tablets three times a day) was added to clear toxins from the liver, and Skin Balance was reduced (to 2 tablets three times a day), as he was having fewer problems with hives and constipation.

Case #5

Rachel, a thirty-five-year-old cook, complained of hives that were particularly severe during the summer. She reported that spicy foods seemed to exacerbate the condition. Traditional Chinese medicine diagnosis revealed that although her pulse was thin and slow, her tongue was red and dry, indicating the presence of heat.

We recommended that she increase her water intake, avoid spicy foods, and take Coptis Purge Fire for one week (3 tablets three times a day). A week later the hives were gone. We reiterated the suggestion that she continue to avoid spicy foods, reduce her intake of alcohol, dairy, and fried foods, and that she increase her intake of vegetables. We also asked her to take Astra Essence (3 tablets three times a day) to nourish yin and tonify qi.

We next saw Rachel six months later when she had another outbreak of hives after eating Thai food. She reported that as long as she took Astra Essence and abstained from spicy food, the hives were controlled. At this point her pulse was normal, and her tongue was red and dry. We suggested that she again take Coptis Purge Fire (3 tablets three times a day) and adhere to the dietary restrictions mentioned above. Once the hives had cleared, we recommended using Nine Flavor Tea (3 tablets three times a day) as a maintenance formula.

Case #6

Marjorie, a thirty-six-year-old waitress, had hives in addition to allergies that caused nasal congestion. She was a smoker and consumed a diet high in sweets, greasy foods, and alcohol. Traditional Chinese medicine diagnosis revealed that her pulse was wiry, and her tongue was red and dry.

We suggested the formulas Xanthium Relieve Surface (3 tablets three times a day) and Coptis Purge Fire (1 tablet three times a day). We also urged Marjorie to go on the Digestive Clearing Program (See Appendix), and to try acupuncture for smoking cessation. She was also told to try irrigating her sinuses twice a day with salt water using a bulb syringe. After two weeks Marjorie noticed little improvement. We asked her if she was able to stick to the diet. She replied that she had tried it for a few days but had become discouraged. She also said she had trouble taking the third dose of Xanthium Relieve Surface. Her tongue and pulse were unchanged. We reiterated that it was important that she follow the diet for two weeks in order to gauge dietary factors contributing to the hives. She was also told to try taking

127

the third dose of Xanthium Relieve Surface with a meal if she was unable to take them on an empty stomach.

Marjorie returned two weeks later with slight improvement in the nasal congestion, but none with the hives. Her pulse was wiry, and her tongue was still red and dry. Other than reducing her dairy intake she had been unable to follow the diet: she had continued to smoke, drink alcohol and diet soft drinks, and eat fried foods and sweets. We suggested she try an aromatherapy compress for the hives, and told her that unless she changed her diet and stopped smoking, treating the hives might not be possible. She did not return for another visit.

Discussion: Hives are often an expression of toxins within the body. In Marjorie's case the toxins were from a combination of smoking, drinking alcohol and diet sodas, and consuming dairy products. Overindulgence in sweets can lead to damp-heat, which in turn can cause stagnation. Dairy foods can cause stagnation, which turns into heat. When too much stagnant heat traps toxins within the body, the body's normal means of eliminating toxins becomes blocked, so the body uses the skin as an alternate route of elimination. Although some people obtain positive results from herbal therapy despite a continued poor diet, the combination of toxins from smoking and dietary factors made this case particularly vexing.

Impetigo

Impetigo is a highly contagious bacterial infection that occurs most often in children. The infection produces blisters that break and release a yellow fluid, which dries to form a honey-colored crust. The standard treatment is oral and topical antibiotics. By using antibacterial soap at home and by seeking early treatment, it may be possible to prevent impetigo from being passed to others.

Undergarments, bedding, towels, and washcloths should be laundered in hot water with bleach. Children should be kept out of daycare or school until the infection clears.

Self-Treatment

◆ Lavender essential oil may be applied after washing thoroughly with antibacterial soap. Dab 2 drops of lavender essential oil on each blister with a cotton swab, making certain to change swabs after each blister. Apply 3 to 4 times daily.

Professional Treatments

◆ Resinall K may be applied after washing thoroughly with antibacterial soap. To prevent cross contamination, pour some Resinall K into a small container first. Then use a cotton swab to dab enough of the formula to cover each blister. Using this method is especially important if multiple family members have impetigo.

◆ Lavender essential oil: Mix 1 part lavender essential oil with 1 part Resinall K. Apply (1 to 2 times daily) after washing thoroughly with antibacterial soap.

Case Study

Larry, a six-year-old, had contracted impetigo at school. Medications did not appear to be effective because of the high reinfection rate among the students. We recommended to his mother that Resinall K be applied topically three times daily, and stressed the importance of frequent hand-washing for Larry, as well as for everyone in the family. Results were seen in one week, with the skin lesions all but gone in two weeks.

Insect Bites

Insect bites may cause itchy red bumps or red ulcerating sores. Most insect bites are self-limiting and resolve in a matter of days. Applying ice or calamine lotion can soothe the itching and inflammation caused by mild insect bites.

If the venom injected into the skin is potent enough, or if a person is hypersensitive to bites, the whole body may become seriously affected. If you, a family member, or a friend develops a swollen face, muscle cramping, breathing problems, headache, nausea, fever, or fainting after being bitten by an insect, seek medical attention immediately. Physicians treat more severe reactions with antihistamines, corticosteriods, and injections such as antivenom.

Self-Treatments

- White or green clay (available in health food stores): Sprinkle on the bite. Apply 2 drops lavender essential oil to make a paste; use 2 to 3 times daily or as needed. If clay is not available, then use lavender essential oil alone (2 drops), 2 to 3 times daily or as needed.
- Activated charcoal: Break open a capsule and sprinkle enough to cover the bite. Cover with an adhesive strip, and keep on for a day.

Professional Treatment

◆ Clear Heat: Crush 3 tablets and mix with water and lavender essential oil (3 to 6 drops, added before the water) to form a paste. Apply topically 4 to 6 times per day.

Jock Itch

Jock itch is known medically as tinea cruris. It is a superficial infection caused primarily by a dermatophyte, a fungus that is parasitic upon the skin. Another fungus, candida, can also cause jock itch. Men are mainly affected, although women can also have the condition, especially those who are obese. The upper thigh and groin are usually involved, with the scrotum being unaffected in men. Signs and symptoms include severe itching, a raised or swollen red, ringed rash with a distinct border and clearing in the center of the rash. Other skin conditions can mimic tinea cruris; therefore, it is important to seek medical attention before trying any self-treatment. Jock itch is treated biomedically with topical antifungal medications.

Self-Treatments

◆ Fungi thrive in warm, moist environments. Wearing loose-fitting underwear and pants during the day, and refraining from wearing underwear or pajamas at night can prevent the genital and groin area from becoming overheated, making it more difficult for a fungal infection to persist.

◆ Dry the affected area thoroughly after showering.

- Topical tea tree oil: Fungal infections often respond to this remedy (follow label directions). However, response time is usually slower than with standard biomedical treatments.
- Oregano essential oil and citrus seed essential oil: Both have antibacterial and antifungal properties. Apply either oil 3 to 4 times daily. If irritation occurs, dilute in water.
- See "Tinea" section for further strategies.

Professional Treatments

- Anti-yeast therapy. (See "Tinea" section.)
- Biocidin: Mix a few drops with 2 oz water. Apply as a cool compress 3 times daily.
- Vagistatin: Mix the contents of 2 to 3 capsules with water or Resinall K (add drop by drop) to make a thin paste. Apply topically 3 times daily.

Kaposi's Sarcoma

Kaposi's sarcoma (KS) usually occurs only in the presence of HIV infection. It is a skin cancer characterized by reddish-purple lesions on the skin, or in the lungs, gastrointestinal tract, spleen, heart, or lymph nodes, and is often accompanied by fatigue, poor appetite, and digestive problems. Standard biomedical treatments include surgery, freezing (cryotherapy), chemotherapy, radiation, and interferon.

Professional Treatments

♦ Resinall K: Apply topically to lesions that have been freshly cleaned. It can also be massaged into painful areas. Resinall K may be used at full strength for small areas, or 1 part Resinall K can be mixed with 3 parts safflower oil for larger areas. If the affected limbs are also cold, make a wash with one-half to 1 cup of cinnamon tea (1 tsp cinnamon powder in 8 oz of water) mixed with 1 dropperful of Resinall K.

♦ Pseudoginseng root (*san qi*): Grind enough to make 500 mg of powder. Mix with 1 tsp water and 1 dropperful of Resinall K to form a paste. Apply to the cleaned lesions 3 times daily.

Leg Ulcers

Leg ulcers are open sores affecting the lower part of the leg. Typically, they begin with itching and pain, followed by swelling, breaking of the skin, oozing of pus, and finally ulcer formation. There may be burning pain, and a foul smell may emanate from the area. Leg ulcers are most commonly caused by poor circulation or by diseases affecting the veins. They may be associated with diabetes, varicose veins, hypertension, rheumatoid arthritis, sickle cell anemia, tumors, infection, contact dermatitis or other disorders, so it is important to see a physician for a definitive diagnosis.

Self-Treatments

♦ Vitamin E topically and internally: Break open capsule and apply topically 2 to 3 times daily; take 400 to 800 IU orally per day.

- Vitamin A topically and internally: Apply topically 2 to 3 times daily; take 10,000 IU orally per day. Vitamin A should be used cautiously during pregnancy; consult your health-care professional about dosages over 5,000 IU.
- Zinc and other antioxidants: Take orally (follow label directions). Zinc is an essential element for wound healing.
- Blueberries, bilberries, or blackberries: Eating 1 cup daily may help improve the integrity of capillaries, and speed healing.

Professional Treatments

- Cir-Q (1 to 2 tablets three times a day) plus Flavonex (3 tablets three times a day).
- Resinall K: Apply topically 3 times daily after thoroughly cleaning the affected area.
- Make a topical wash by combining equal parts pseudoginseng root *(san qi)*, safflower *(hong hua)*, sparganium *(san leng)*, and honeysuckle flower *(jin yin hua)*. Simmer herbs for twenty minutes, strain, and repeat, combining both mixtures.

Case Study

Doug, seventy-five-years-old, had developed a leg ulcer because of poor circulation. The ulcer was deep to the bone, and about the diameter of two quarters. He was prescribed antibiotics by his physician; however, the ulcer was unresponsive. Doug also had other signs of poor circulation, such as cold feet and hands. Traditional Chinese medicine diagnosis revealed that his pulse was weak and slow, and his tongue pale.

To promote better circulation, we recommended topical and oral herbs. The formula Flavonex (3 tablets three times a day) was suggested as an overall tonifier and to improve circulation. Resinall K was applied twice daily to the ulcer after cleansing and disinfecting it. We also had Doug use the following formula as a hot herbal soak twice a day: coptis (*huang lian*), scute (*huang qin*), pseudoginseng (*san qi*), salvia (*dang shen*), and carthamus (*hong hua*). After two months on this protocol, the size of the ulcer was reduced by about half. Within six months all that remained of the ulcer was a scar.

Diabetic Foot Care

One of the complications of diabetes is damage to the nerves and small blood vessels. The feet are particularly vulnerable and ulcers can result if precautions are not taken. Wash them daily in warm water, and dry them thoroughly. Check your feet daily for cuts, blisters, and swelling. Protect your feet with socks and shoes that breathe, and wear slippers in the house. Exercise everyday, and keep your feet up while sitting. Call your health professional if any foot problem develops. For further information a free booklet, "Take Care of Your Feet for a Lifetime," is available from NIH, 800-438-5383. Ask for publication #98-4285.

Lice (Pediculosis)

Lice are tiny parasitic insects spread through direct contact with an infected person's hair, or personal items such as brushes, combs, hats, or towels. There are three species of lice: head lice, pubic lice (crabs), and body lice. Head lice are very prevalent in schools and daycare centers. The main symptoms of lice infestation are intense itching from the insect bites. Scratch marks are often present, which may become infected.

Over-the-counter or prescription medications such as Lindane and Permethrin may be applied. Sheets and towels should be soaked in bleach and then washed thoroughly in very hot water, or these articles should be incinerated. Hats, combs, and brushes should be thrown away. Sexual partners of those with pubic lice should be examined and treated.

(Lindane is banned in California, as it is a nerve toxin leading to many side effects. Shampoos and creams with Lindane when rinsed off pollute the water supply.)

Self-Treatments

♦ Thyme oil: Thyme is a natural insecticide. Add 3 to 4 drops to 1 tablespoon of shampoo, mix well and apply to the scalp and hair for five minutes before rinsing with warm water. Apply 1 to 2 times daily.

♦ Vinegar remedy: Mix equal parts of warm water and vinegar and apply to the scalp. Then cover with a shower cap. Remove cap after fifteen minutes and rinse hair. Apply once daily.

♦ For body lice: Mix 2 drops each of thyme essential oil, cypress essential oil, and eucalyptus essential oil with 1 tablespoon of safflower oil (increase amounts proportionally if necessary). Apply over entire body 3 times daily.

Professional Treatments

♦ Chaparral wash: Mix 1 tsp chaparral powder with 8 to 16 oz water. Apply to affected area or wash scalp and hair with the preparation.

♦ Cir-Q topically: Crush 2 tablets, combine with 8 oz water, simmer for 2 minutes. Allow to cool and then apply to affected area. Apply 2 times daily.

Case Study

Elliot, a twenty-five-year-old teacher, contracted drug-resistant body lice from his partner who worked in a daycare center. Traditional Chinese medicine diagnosis revealed that his pulse was slightly slow and his tongue looked normal.

We recommended Cir-Q topically (2 applications per day—morning and night—to cover his entire body). After one week, Elliot felt that the itching was greatly reduced; however, the lice had not been totally eliminated because he still experienced itching at night. We suggested he alternate the Cir-Q wash with a chaparral wash. One week later, he reported that the lice were totally eliminated.

Lichen Planus

Lichen planus is an itchy rash characterized by reddish-purple spots on the skin. Onset can be sudden or occur over a period of months. The lesions are usually found symmetrically on both sides of the body, on the insides of the wrists or the backs of the legs. About half of the patients have lesions in the mouth or other mucous membranes, such as the vaginal or rectal area. Dryness and a metallic or burning sensation in the mouth may be the first sign of this condition. Flare-ups may last up to several months. Though the cause of this condition is unknown, it is thought that flare-ups are related to stress. Biomedical treatment involves using topical corticosteroid medications for lesions that are limited, and systemic corticosteroids for more severe cases.

Professional Treatments

- Skin Balance (2 to 3 tablets three or four times a day): Use for severe itching. Reduce dosage if diarrhea results.
- Coptis Purge Fire with Skin Balance (2 tablets each four times a day): Use for oral lesions. Reduce dosages if diarrhea results.
- Resinall K: Apply to lesions to reduce itching and speed healing.

Case Study

Arlette, a thirty-two-year-old manager, had lichen planus for the past year. It had come about after a long period of eighty-hour work weeks. All tests were negative for any other conditions. She had an itchy rash on her scalp and the insides of her wrists, and whitish plaques inside her mouth and vagina. Her nails were brittle and starting to show pitting. Her skin in general was dry. Other symptoms included exhaustion, low back pain, and hives that were triggered by exposure to cold. Traditional Chinese medicine diagnosis revealed that her pulse was weak and deep, and her tongue was red and dry.

We recommended the formula Marrow Plus (3 tablets four times a day) to nourish the blood. Arlette was also asked to apply Resinall K topically diluted in safflower oil. We suggested a high-potency fish oil supplement (2 capsules with each meal), as well as eating fatty fish and using flaxseed oil on vegetables and salads. She was also referred for acupuncture to help relieve stress and boost the immune system. Within one month, Arlette experienced some improvement. Her skin was less dry and itchy, and her pulse was stronger and her tongue was less red and moister. She continued on the protocol for three months, showing gradual improvement of all her symptoms.

Lupus

Lupus is a condition of chronic inflammation of the connective tissue. The more common form of lupus is called discoid lupus erythematosus (DLE), while the more serious form is known as systemic lupus erythematosus (SLE). DLE rash begins as red, round thickened or scaling areas that usually appear on the face, nose, or scalp, or behind the ears. DLE affecting the scalp may cause hair loss. In the initial stages of SLE, an identical rash can occur, or a red butterfly-shaped rash may appear over the cheeks and bridge of the nose. Since the skin lesions of DLE and SLE may be identical, a thorough medical evaluation is necessary to determine if systemic involvement is present.

In addition to skin lesions, SLE typically involves joint inflammation and may lead to increased sensitivity to sun exposure and increased susceptibility to infection, fever, fatigue, poor digestion, ulcers in the mouth and nose, vision problems, bleeding problems, edema, depression, anxiety, and swollen lymph nodes. SLE can also affect any organ system, and may cause anemia, neurologic or psychiatric problems, renal failure, pleurisy, arthritis, and pericarditis. A small percentage of people with DLE eventually develop some degree of systemic involvement, sometimes limited solely to joint pain.

SLE is thought to be an inherited autoimmune disorder. It is more prevalent in women and people of Asian or African descent. Stress, infection, childbirth, and sun exposure may cause flare-ups. If you have DLE or SLE, and must go out in the sun, use a sunscreen containing PABA with an SPF of at least 15, wear a hat and sunglasses, and cover your arms and legs. Try to get plenty of sleep in order to allow the body to recover from daily activities and stress. Tiredness and stress wear down the immune system, which can lead to flare-ups. Steroids, immune suppressive medications, and chloroquine are often prescribed.

Self-Treatments

- Antioxidant formula that includes 800 IU vitamin E (follow label directions).
- Gotu kola (2,000 to 4,000 mg daily).
- Fish oil concentrate that contains EPA/DHA: Slowly increase dosage to 3 to 10 grams daily.

Professional Treatments

- Lithospermum 15 (3 tablets four times a day): Use to regulate the immune system during flare-ups.
- Thymus extracts: Use to boost immune function. Follow label directions.
- Thymus shampoo: Use to promote hair growth.
- Astra Isatis (2 tablets four times a day) with Clear Heat (2 tablets four times a day): Use for symptoms of fatigue and fever.
- Astra Isatis with Power Mushrooms (2 tablets each four times a day): Use for fatigue with cold signs.
- Nine Flavor Tea and Clear Heat (2 tablets each four times a day): Use for symptoms of afternoon fever and dryness and ulcers of the mouth.

Case Studies

Case #1

Marjorie, a fifty-year-old woman with discoid lupus was taking prednisone (10 mg per day) and chloroquine, and receiving steroid injections as often as once every two weeks. She was also taking medication for high blood pressure. The problems for which she was seeking help were skin disfigurement and burning sensation, joint pain, headaches, hair loss, fatigue, constipation, and weight gain; she was about sixty pounds overweight. Traditional Chinese medicine diagnosis revealed that her pulse was weak, wiry, and fast, and her tongue was pale with a heavy white coating.

We recommended a decoction of the following herbs: white peony *(bai shao)*, bupleurum *(chai hu)*, raw rehmannia *(sheng di)*, scute *(huang qin)*, alisma *(ze xie)*, abrus *(ji gu cao)*, lonicera *(jin yin hua)*, gentian *(long dan cao)*, jasmine *(su xin hua)*, origanum *(tu xiang ru)*, melia *(chuan lian zi)*, anemarrhena *(zhi mu)*, and sanguisorba *(di yu)*. In addition we recommended the formula Skin Balance (2 tablets three times a day).

Two weeks later Marjorie reported a decrease in the burning sensation, but was worried that a headache she had for three days might be a signal of an imminent flare-up. Her tongue had a thick yellow-white coating, and her pulse was unchanged. We revised her decoction by adding American ginseng *(xi yang shen)*, phellodendron *(huang bai)*, chrysanthemum *(ju hua)*, ophiopogon *(mai men dong)*, scrophularia *(xuan shen)*, lithospermum *(zi cao)*, and eclipta *(han lian cao)*, and omitting sanguisorba *(di yu)*, anemarrhena *(zhi mu)*, melia *(chuan lian zi)*, jasmine *(su xin hua)*, and gentian *(long dan cao)*. In addition, we recommended Clear Heat (2 tablets three times a day) instead of Skin Balance. She was instructed that if her skin burned, she could apply Clear Heat as a poultice.

Three weeks later, Marjorie reported less burning and itching, but was very concerned about hair loss. She pushed aside her hair and showed us a very red bald spot about three inches long by two inches wide. Her pulse was thin and rapid, and her tongue had a heavy white coating. We gave her a new formula consisting of American ginseng *(xi yang shen)*, white peony *(bai shao)*, peony root *(dan pi)*, rehmannia *(sheng di)*, he shou wu *(he shou*

141

wu), alisma *(ze xie),* abrus *(ji gu cao),* chrysanthemum *(ju hua),* cimicifuga *(sheng ma),* origanum *(tu xiang ru),* scrophularia *(xuan shen),* cassia *(jue ming zi),* and lithospermum *(zi cao).* We also asked her to continue taking Clear Heat (2 tablets four times a day).

Three weeks later, Marjorie indicated that her skin felt much better, and she had not had any headaches since her previous visit. However, she said that she did have a flare-up a few days earlier because she was angry and upset that her job was going to be terminated due to corporate restructuring. Her pulse was rapid, weak, and irregular; and her tongue had less white coating than before. We added the herb albizzia *(he huan pi)* to her formula, asked her to continue taking Clear Heat (2 tablets four times a day). We also suggested a thymus shampoo and lotion for her hair loss.

Marjorie returned one month later full of optimism; she had experienced one minor flare-up, but had not required a cortisone injection as was typical in the past. In addition, her headaches were not as frequent or severe, and she thought the thymus preparations were helping her hair loss. Her pulse was fast and weak in the heart and lung positions, and her tongue was pale with a white coating. We recommended she continue taking the herbal decoction and using the thymus preparations. To help keep her calm through her stressful job situation we recommended the formula Kava Seng (1 to 2 tablets two times a day). Clear Heat was discontinued.

In a follow-up appointment several months later, all Marjorie's symptoms had improved so much that she now needed fewer steroid injections, and was looking forward to when she could start tapering off the prednisone. She had begun an exercise routine of working out at the gym three days a week alternating with walking the other three days.

Case #2

Laura, a forty-five-year-old lupus patient, complained of upper body rashes, joint inflammation, fatigue, headaches, recurrent cold sores, indigestion, and constipation. She had these symptoms for three years. Traditional Chinese medicine diagnosis revealed that her pulse was rapid, and her tongue was purple with a yellow-gray patchy coating.

We recommended Mobility 2 (2 tablets four times a day) to reduce dampness and promote blood circulation, and Clear Heat to reduce toxicity (2 tablets four times a day the first week, 3 tablets four times a day thereafter). We also suggested PB 8 acidophilus/bifidus (2 capsules before bed and 2 upon waking). After three weeks, Laura reported improvement in the rash, slightly less joint pain, and fewer headaches. Her pulse was slower, but her tongue was unchanged. She continued on the protocol for another four weeks, with her skin rash improving significantly. The joint pain continued to improve, and her headaches were much less severe. As Laura was having occasional loose stools, we suggested she reduce Clear Heat (to 1 tablet four times a day), and increase Mobility 2 (to 3 tablets four times a day), and continue taking the PB 8 acidophilus/bifidus (at the same dosage). She was also asked to take Colostroplex, a bovine colostrum product (1 tablet per day), to improve her immune and gastrointestinal systems.

After three months on the herbal and supplement protocol, Laura no longer had rashes, headaches, indigestion, cold sores, and constipation. Her joint pain and inflammation were greatly reduced.

Case #3

Lily, thirty-two, was diagnosed with lupus and fibromyalgia. She was on disability as she was suffering from severe fatigue, dizziness, poor concentration, joint and muscle pain, nausea and headaches, and sensitivity to light and heat. She was taking several medications for depression and lupus. Traditional Chinese medicine diagnosis revealed that her pulse was weak and sinking, and her tongue was purplish.

Because Lily's symptoms were worse upon exposure to light and heat, we recommended herbs that nourish yin and clear heat. She was given the formulas Nine Flavor Tea (3 tablets four times a day), which was aimed at replenishing yin and clearing heat, and Lithospermum 15 (3 tablets four times a day), which was for clearing heat and toxin, moving blood, and nourishing yin. After one week she reported that her nausea had increased and she had become bloated after taking the herbs. Apparently, Lily was having difficulty digesting the yin tonics, which are often cloying in nature. Attempting to circumvent this problem, we recommended she take the herbs with meals. After another week she was still having problems digesting the herbs, so we suggested that the dosage be reduced (to 3 times per day). We also had her start on Quiet Digestion (1 tablet four times a day). As Lily was fond of Thai food, we advised her to reduce her intake of spicy foods, and especially to eliminate chili peppers from her diet because spicy foods tend to promote buildup of heat and dampness. We treated Lily for several months. The protocol helped reduce the duration of the flare-ups. All of her symptoms improved including the muscle pain. Her pulse was stronger and her tongue no longer as purple.

Case #4

Mary, forty-four, had been diagnosed with lupus as a teenager. Stress from her job and difficulties with her children brought on a flare-up. Her main symptoms were joint pain, edema, fatigue, depression, sinus congestion, and frequent thirst. Her pulse was slippery and weak, and her tongue was pale and swollen.

We recommended the formulas Drain Dampness to reduce edema and Mobility 2 to increase blood circulation and reduce pain and edema. We instructed her to use 2 tablets of each formula four times a day the first week, and 3 of each four times a day thereafter. After two weeks, the edema and joint pain were improved; however, Mary still felt fatigued and depressed. Her pulse and tongue were unchanged. We suggested she try to exercise every day, and that when she took the herbal tablets she drink several glasses of water and ginger tea. Ginger tea is warming, helps treat joint pain, and helps reduce phlegm. Her pulse and tongue were unchanged.

After four weeks, Mary reported significantly less joint pain and edema. Her fatigue was better, but she remained depressed. Her pulse was less slippery, and her tongue looked less swollen. At this point we recommended the formulas Aspiration (2 to 3 tablets four times a day) for depression, and Rehmannia 8 (2 to 3 tablets four times a day) as a kidney tonic that helps treat edema. Drain Dampness and Mobility 2 were stopped. Mary remained on this protocol for three months with moderate improvements of all symptoms.

Case #5

Sydney, a forty-four-year-old teacher, had several lupus flare-ups each year during stressful times. She also reported fatigue, thirst, and occasional night sweats. Her complexion was slightly pale.

Sydney was taking prednisone and Plaquenil and came to us seeking immune supportive herbs. Traditional Chinese medicine diagnosis revealed that her pulse was sinking, slightly rapid, and deficient in the kidney positions, and her tongue was red and dry.

In addition to protecting herself from the sun, we recommended that Sydney nourish the yin by increasing her consumption of fruits and vegetables and by drinking at least 64 oz of water daily. Since she was not having a flare-up at the time, we suggested Astra Isatis (2 tablets four times a day) to support the immune system, clear toxins, and to tonify yin and yang. She was also given Nine Flavor Tea (2 tablets four times a day) to nourish yin.

After following this protocol for three months, Sydney reported increased energy and a reduction of night sweats, and no flare-ups of lupus. She was able to reduce the prednisone from 20 mg to 5 mg daily. She remained on the Plaquenil.

Case #6

Cindy, a forty-three-year-old lawyer, consulted our clinic for lupus. She had skin lesions, joint pain, fatigue, and dry mouth and eyes. She took Naprosyn for pain, and covered her skin with hypoallergenic makeup to disguise the skin lesions. She generally felt hotter than other people, especially in the afternoon. Therefore, it was not unusual that she drank a lot of water because she was constantly thirsty. Traditional Chinese medicine diagnosis revealed that her pulse was thin and wiry, and her tongue was red and dry.

We recommended Nine Flavor Tea (3 tablets three times a day) to nourish yin, and Clear Heat (2 tablets three times a day) to reduce toxins and heat. We also suggested White Flower Oil to be used topically for joint pain, with heat signs. After three weeks Cindy indicated that there was slight improvement, although she was taking the herbs only twice rather than three times per day. We encouraged her to take the full dosage of herbs, and to also take the herb Smilax (1 teaspoon two times a day) with the tablets to further reduce heat and toxicity. After two weeks there was improvement in all signs and symptoms. After remaining on the protocol for three months, Cindy exhibited fewer signs of heat, and thus continued to take Nine Flavor Tea (3 tablets three times a day) but used the Clear Heat and Smilax only as needed. Her mouth and eyes were no longer dry and her joint pain was greatly diminished.

Case #7

Carrie, a seventeen-year-old student, was recently diagnosed with lupus. Her main symptoms were joint pain and swelling, fatigue, swollen glands, mouth sores, and occasional dizziness. She was on Plaquenil and prednisone. Traditional Chinese medicine diagnosis revealed that her pulse was thin and slow and her tongue purple.

We recommended a combination of Mobility 3 (2 tablets four times a day) to help relieve joint pain and tonify qi, and Astra Isatis (2 tablets four times a day) to tonify qi and to clear heat and toxins. Additionally, we suggested she take 1 to 3 teaspoons of cod liver oil per day for its essential fatty acids, which help reduce inflammation. Two weeks later Carrie indicated that she felt better, though her pulse and tongue were unchanged. After remaining on the protocol for another month she reported less joint swelling and pain, improvement in the fatigue and swollen glands, and complete resolution of the mouth sores. Despite these improvements her pulse was still slow and thin, and her tongue was reddish-purple, manifestations that we attributed to a weak constitution.

147

Carrie continued on this protocol for three months, at which point she came down with a cold and was given Isatis Gold and Nasal Tabs (2 tablets of each four times a day). Once these symptoms were resolved, she was placed back on the initial protocol. As winter approached and the weather grew colder, Carrie's joint pain worsened. To help alleviate the pain we recommended that she take the herbal tablets with tea made with powdered ginger. Carrie remained on the protocol and experienced less joint pain, improved energy, and resolution of the swollen glands. Her mouth sores also did not recur.

Lymphedema

Lymphedema is swelling of a limb caused by abnormal accumulation of lymph. This can be due to blockage, damage, or removal of the lymph vessels or nodes so that drainage of lymph is disrupted. Diseases such as filariasis, a parasitic disease of the tropics, causes lymphedema when small worms block the lymph passages. Blockage may also occur when cancer spreads through the lymphatic system and settles in the lymph vessels. Surgical removal of the lymph nodes, particularly of the underarm area during cancer assessment and treatment often results in lymphedema.

Biomedical treatment usually involves measures such as massaging the affected limb, wearing a compression sleeve, taking diuretic medications, or exercises with the arm or leg elevated. When the lymphedema is long-standing and the limb becomes so large that it causes disability, surgery can be performed to remove the extra tissue and skin.

Self-Treatments

- High-potency bromelain (500 mg daily) taken alone. Or for higher efficacy, take in a formula that contains other bromelain with proteolytic enzymes.
- Incorporating seaweed into the diet may also be helpful.

Professional Treatments

- Bupleurum Entangled Qi (BEQ) is especially useful for lymphedema affected by the underarms and breast area. Take 3 tablets a day between meals.
- Resinall E: Use for pain and swelling (2 to 3 tablets, three to four times a day between meals).
- Clear Heat (3 tablets four times a day): Use for heat signs.
- Formula V contains horse chestnut seed extract and supportive herbs that help treat lymphedema. Take 1 to 2 tablets three times a day.
- Clear Phlegm (2 to 3 tablets four times a day): Use to clear sluggish lymph by promoting the flow of lymph. Discontinue or reduce dosage if dryness of the mouth is noticed. May be combined with Clear Heat, Resinall E, or Formula V.

Case Study

Rosemary, thirty-eight, had developed swollen and painful lymph nodes following breast cancer surgery, during which the axillary lymph nodes were removed. She appeared tired and had very dark circles under the eyes. Traditional Chinese medicine diagnosis revealed that her pulse was thin and slow, and her tongue was red with a thick, yellow-gray coating.

We recommended Bupleurum Entangled Qi (3 tablets four times a day) to promote blood circulation and to eliminate the phlegm that was manifested by the thick tongue coating. We also suggested she drink three cups a day of dandelion tea, which has detoxifying properties and is specific for breast disease. In addition, we advised her to eat seaweed to remove toxins from the lymph system.

After three weeks, Rosemary reported greater energy and a decrease in the lymph node swelling and pain. Her pulse was unchanged, although the tongue coating was thinner. We added the formula Six Gentlemen (2 tablets four times a day) to her protocol to tonify qi and to further boost her energy. Six Gentlemen also contains herbs for phlegm and dampness to support the herbs in Bupleurum Entangled Qi to reduce the edema.

One month later, Rosemary experienced even further reduction of lymph node swelling and pain, and her energy had improved. She wanted to discontinue all herbs, but we suggested she stay on a maintenance dose of Bupleurum Entangled Qi (3 tablets three times a day) to assist her circulation and thereby improve the lymphatic system's ability to clear toxins from the body. We also encouraged her to start a stress reduction and exercise program.

Measles

Measles is a highly contagious disease caused by a virus that is spread through airborne droplets from the nose, throat, and mouth of an infected person. Measles is most contagious during the incubation period of nine to eleven days before symptoms appear. One episode usually confers lifelong immunity.

Measles begins as a fever with coughing, sneezing, and sore throat. After one to seven days a red rash appears on the face and behind the ears, and then spreads to cover the entire body. In addition, there may be swollen eyelids and white spots inside the lining of the cheeks.

The standard biomedical treatment for measles includes rest, Tylenol or other aspirin substitutes, and cough medicine. Antibiotics may be recommended if a bacterial infection such as pneumonia develops. If you or your child develops measles, see a health professional to rule out other diseases such as German measles (rubella), scarlet fever, drug rashes, Rocky Mountain Spotted fever, and other viral infections.

Vaccination is recommended at fifteen months and at about twelve years of age. Individuals who should not receive vaccination include those who have a fever, those who have already had measles, and those with weak immune systems.

Self-Treatments

- Zinc lozenges (45 to 60 mg a day for adults; 30 mg for adolescents; 15 to 20 mg for young children).
- Cod liver oil internally (1 to 3 tbsp daily).
- Decoction of cherry pits: Decoct 9 g crushed cherry pits in 32 oz water for 20 to 30 minutes until 6 oz of fluid remains. Strain and discard the dregs. Take one decoction daily until the rash vents (begins to fade). To make a sponge bath, decoct one-third pound (150 g) of crushed cherry pits, and apply lukewarm 1 to 2 times daily.

Professional Treatments

The following treatments may shorten the duration of the measles episode. For the initial stage of fever, runny nose, cough, and a floating, rapid pulse, the following are suggested:

- For children, use Yin Chao Jin (1 to 2 tablets per 10 lbs body-weight per day); or use Yin Chao Junior (1 to 3 dropperfuls, 4 to 6 times per day).
- For adults, use Yin Chao Jin (1 to 3 tablets, 4 to 6 times per day).

For fever, thirst, irritability, redness of the eyes, cough, and difficulty sleeping, the following are suggested:

- For children use Coptis Purge Fire and Clear Heat (1 tablet per day of each formula per 10 lbs of bodyweight).
- For adults use Coptis Purge Fire and Clear Heat (2 tablets each, 4 to 6 times per day).
- Chaparral compress: Mix 1 tsp of chaparral powder with 8 oz boiling water. Steep for 15 minutes, strain, and apply as a cool compress.

Nail Fungus

Fungal infections of the nails are stubborn conditions that are difficult to treat. The cause is usually the same species of fungus that gives rise to ringworm. The toenails are more often affected than the fingernails. Symptoms include thickened and yellow or white nails that are lusterless. Left untreated the nail eventually separates from the nail bed and falls off.

Biomedical treatment involves oral antifungal medications such as itraconazole (Sporanox) or terbinafine (Lamisil). These medications have a cure rate of about seventy to eighty percent, and are very expensive. The fungus may recur once the medications are stopped. Continual use of the medications may lead to liver damage. Some dermatologists remove the entire nail and then prescribe topical antifungal medication. Typically the herbal treatments below take up to six months to work.

Self-Treatments

◆ Citrus seed oil (1 to 2 times daily): Apply directly to nail and nail bed. Or, for better efficacy, soak foot in bath first. Put 10 drops in a basin of warm water and soak the affected foot 15 to 20 minutes. After thoroughly drying the foot and affected nail, apply 1 or 2 drops directly to the nail and nail bed. Oregano oil may be used as a substitute, or can be added.

◆ Tea tree oil: Apply directly to the nail and nail bed (1 to 2 times daily).

Professional Treatments

◆ Antifungal therapy: Clean affected area well with soap and water. Apply 1 to 2 drops undiluted hydrogen peroxide to the nail and nail bed, and leave on for one minute. Dry well. Apply oregano oil or tea tree oil followed by DMSO. DMSO helps facilitate absorption of the herbal oil through the nail.

◆ Biocidin: Apply 2 to 3 drops directly to the affected area (1 to 2 times daily). If irritation of the nail develops, mix 1 part Biocidin with 4 parts olive oil, then apply. As a soak, put 5 drops Biocidin in a basin filled with 1 quart of hot water. Soak for 15 minutes, 1 to 2 times daily.

Pityriasis Rosea

Pityriasis rosea means "red scaling." This condition usually affects young adults. Its cause is unknown, although viral infection is suspected. The first sign of this condition is a one to three-inch pink lesion, known as the herald patch, on the torso. Several days to weeks later more patches appear on the trunk, upper arms and legs, sometimes in a Christmas tree pattern. The face, hands, and feet are usually not involved. Typically, other than some itching, there is no discomfort. It is important to have a medical evaluation to rule out more serious diseases that cause a similar rash.

Pityriasis rosea is a self-limiting condition that runs its course in four to six weeks. Standard biomedical treatments include lubricants, anti-itch creams, and cortisone creams or oral medications.

Self-Treatments

- For itching, mix 5 drops lavender essential oil with 1 tbsp olive or safflower oil. Apply 2 to 3 times daily.
- Take an essential fatty acid (EFA) formula, such as cod liver oil, which contains both EPA and DHA (3 to 10 g daily, or 1 to 3 tsp daily).

Professional Treatments

- Skin Balance (2 to 3 tablets three or four times a day).
  - For heat signs, add Clear Heat (1 to 2 tablets three or four times a day).
  - For dampness and poor circulation, add Mobility 2 (2 to 3 three or four times a day).
- For redness and swelling, use Clear Heat and/or Coptis Purge Fire (2 tablets each four times a day).

Pityriasis Rubra Pilaris

Pityriasis rubra pilaris (PRP) is a rare chronic skin disease that is frequently mistaken for another condition, usually psoriasis. PRP is characterized by redness, scaling, and thickening of the skin. Orange-red (salmon-colored) scaly patches can involve large portions of the body or just the elbows and knees. PRP can be an inherited condition, with onset in childhood. Or more often, the onset occurs for unknown reasons in adulthood, usually in the forties. The patches usually start on the scalp, face, or chest, and then extend downward, often involving the entire body. The clinical hallmarks of PRP are the small islands of unaffected skin, and thickened palms and soles which develop as the condition progresses. Itching is quite severe initially, and becomes more bearable as time goes on. Biomedical treatment involves using topical corticosteroids, retinoids, and as a last resort, methotrexate. But because such treatment is not always effective, alternative modalities such as herbs may be helpful.

Self-Treatments

- ◆ For itching, mix 5 drops lavender essential oil with 1 tbsp olive or safflower oil. Apply 2 to 3 times daily.
- ◆ Fish oil that contains EPA and DHA: Use to help resolve the scaly patches (3 to 10 g daily).

Professional Treatments

- ◆ Skin Balance (2 to 3 tablets three or four times a day).
  - ▪ For excess heat, add Clear Heat (1 to 3 tablets three or four times a day).
  - ▪ For itching due to blood deficiency, add Marrow Plus (2 to 3 tablets three or four times a day).
  - ▪ For yin deficiency, add Nine Flavor Tea (2 tablets three or four times a day).

155

◆ Resinall K: Use topically for scaly patches (apply three to four times daily).

Case Study

Kyle, a forty-eight-year-old computer professional, came to our clinic complaining of pityriasis rubra pilaris. He had red itchy skin surrounding the hair follicles over his entire body. He was experiencing a "pins and needles" pain, and his palms and soles were thick. He also complained of insomnia, constipation, and intestinal gas. He had prostatitis, which was causing a burning sensation during urination and a chronic sinus infection that was producing thick green nasal discharge. Kyle had tried a zinc preparation for his skin, but when that was unsuccessful, his doctor switched him to Retin-A, which he was currently on. He had been treated with repeat rounds of antibiotics for his prostatitis, and had even tried saw palmetto, but neither had helped. His pulse was wiry and weak, and his tongue was purple.

We recommended Kyle start on Skin Balance (3 tablets three times a day), and Quiet Digestion (2 tablets three times a day). We also suggested he take a fish oil mixture containing high-potency EPA and DHA (6 capsules daily), and flaxseed oil (1 tbsp daily) on salads or vegetables. After one week, Kyle reported his skin felt slightly less itchy, and his prostate felt better. His pulse was still wiry and weak, and his tongue was still purple. At this time, we asked if he had tried to eliminate some foods from his diet to see whether any particular items were affecting his health. Kyle indicated that he had done so, but no food item stood out. We then suggested he increase the dosage of Skin Balance (to 4 tablets three times a day) and the amount of flaxseed oil (to 2 tbsp daily). He continued the Quiet Digestion and fish oil as before.

We saw Kyle three weeks later. His itching was reduced and

his skin was noticeably less red. He indicated that he was experiencing less burning due to the prostatitis. The nasal discharge was now less thick and green. His constipation had improved and he was having bowel movements every two days instead of the every four days when we first saw him. His pulse was less wiry, and his tongue was less purple. We recommended that he add black currant oil (6 capsules daily) to his protocol. As of this writing, we continue to work with Kyle to reduce his symptoms.

Prickly Heat Rash (Miliaria Rubra)

Prickly heat rash is characterized by pin-sized bumps surrounded by a patch of red skin, and is usually found in areas where sweat accumulates, typically on the neck, chest, groin, and armpits. Prickly heat rash develops when sweat is unable to reach the skin's surface to evaporate. Instead, it becomes trapped below the surface of the skin where it can cause an irritating prickling sensation and severe itching.

Treatment includes keeping the affected areas cool and dry, and wearing clean, loose-fitting, starch-free clothing to facilitate sweat evaporation. Frequent cold showers or sponging of the affected areas may help alleviate itching. After showering, dry the affected areas thoroughly and apply calamine lotion.

Self-Treatments

- Peppermint tea: Apply as a soak. Or, a moistened peppermint tea bag may be applied to the affected areas or used in a bath.
- Cucumber-lemon soak: Put 1 to 2 half-inch slices of peeled, fresh cucumber or a half-inch slice of lemon in 8 oz water;

157

allow to steep for 45 to 60 minutes. Apply liquid with a wash-cloth to affected area (2 to 3 times daily).

- ◆ Fresh cucumber slices: Apply to the affected areas (15 to 20 minutes, 2 to 3 times daily).
- ◆ Stay well hydrated by drinking at least 64 ounces of water daily.
- ◆ Increase your intake of fresh fruits and vegetables.
- ◆ Vitamin E (400 to 800 IU daily).
- ◆ Lavender and chamomile remedy: Add 2 drops of lavender essential oil to 4 oz chamomile tea. Use a cotton ball to dab the mixture on the affected areas (2 to 3 times daily); or use a washcloth and apply as a cool compress to the affected areas (2 to 3 times daily). Or, one part of this mixture may be added to one part aloe gel and applied to the affected areas (2 to 3 times daily).

Professional Treatments

- ◆ Nine Flavor Tea (3 to 4 tablets four times a day): Use for persistent heat rash with afternoon fever, thirst, and dry throat. For severe heat signs, add Coptis Purge Fire (1 to 2 tablets, 3 to 4 times per day; also apply topically as a soak).

Case Study

Virginia, a thirty-eight-year-old teacher, was affected by prickly heat rash with weeping sores every summer. When she came to our clinic, she was in the middle of such an episode. She had no other symptoms. Her doctor had prescribed an antibiotic ointment to prevent infection of the sores. Traditional Chinese medicine diagnosis revealed that her pulse was wiry and her tongue was red.

We recommended cleaning the affected areas twice daily with soap and water and then submerging them in a Coptis Purge Fire soak. She continued using the antibiotic ointment following the herbal soak. After one week Virginia called to say the rash had completely resolved. She stopped taking the herbs except when she felt the rash coming on; when used at that stage the herbs have a preventive effect. We suggested she take Nine Flavor Tea to address the constitutional yin deficiency that made her susceptible to prickly heat rash, but she was not inclined to take herbs on an ongoing basis.

Psoriasis

Psoriasis is characterized by elevated, red, and inflamed patches, which are often covered by silvery scales. The patches are usually asymptomatic, except during flare-ups when itching and a burning sensation may be present. Psoriasis can be found anywhere on the body, though typically the knees, elbows, and scalp are affected. Fingernails can show yellowing, with stippling and pitting of the nail bed. With psoriatic arthritis, there may be joint pain and stiffness. A skin biopsy may be done to confirm a visual diagnosis. Medical attention should be sought immediately if psoriasis develops over a large portion of the body.

The biomedical cause of psoriasis appears to be an autoimmune phenomenon. Also, persons with psoriasis often have a family history for the disease. Flare-ups of psoriasis can be triggered by emotional stress, skin damage, cold weather, physical illness, or other factors. Medications such as lithium, quinidine, and those that treat high blood pressure and inflammation are also known to exacerbate psoriasis.

Biomedical treatment of psoriasis involves topical agents when the affected areas are limited to less than twenty percent of body surface. Such agents used include emollients, keratolytics, corticosteroids, coal tar, among others. Systemic and more aggressive treatment is used for psoriasis that covers more than twenty percent of the body surface. Such treatment involves phototherapy and medications such as retinoids (Acitretin), antimetabolites (Methotrexate), and calcineurin inhibitors (Cyclosporin). Side effects are often associated with long-term administration of all medications, whether topical or systemic. For example, corticosteroids often become ineffective and may exacerbate psoriasis by masking symptoms.

Psoriasis can be a debilitating disease physically and emotionally because of the unsightly blemishes. Therefore, complementary therapies such as acupuncture, meditation, and yoga may be helpful. An elimination diet may get to the root of the problem, since there appears to be anecdotal evidence that diet and nutrition are causal factors for psoriasis flare-ups (see Digestive Clearing Plan, Appendix A).

Self-Treatments

- ◆ Oatmeal baths: Use to soothe psoriatic areas (follow label directions).
- ◆ Black currant oil (3,000 mg daily).
- ◆ Pine tar soap (follow label directions).
- ◆ Zinc and other antioxidant supplements with multimineral ingredients (follow label directions).
- ◆ Smilax (sarsaparilla) (one-half to 1 tsp three times a day; reduce dosage if diarrhea occurs).
- ◆ Flaxseed oil (1 to 3 tbsp daily) taken with vitamin E (400 to 800 IU daily), or fish oil concentrate (3 to 10 g daily).

Professional Treatments

- Skin Balance (2 to 3 tablets, 3 to 4 times daily).
  - For heat signs add Clear Heat (1 to 2 tablets three times a day).
  - For dryness add Marrow Plus (2 to 3 tablets four times a day).
- Mobility 2 (3 tablets, 3 to 4 times daily): Use for swollen joints.
- Zaocys tablets (3 tablets, 3 to 4 times daily) for psoriatic arthritis.
- Resinall K: Apply undiluted directly to affected areas (1 to 3 times daily); if skin is too sensitive to undiluted Resinall K, then dilute 1 part Resinall K with 3 parts safflower or avocado oil and apply to affected areas (1 to 3 times daily).
- Dictamus (3 tablets, 3 to 4 times daily): Use for cases with more scaling and itching, and less redness and heat signs. (If heat signs are more prominent, use Skin Balance as above.)

Case Studies

Case #1

Steve, a fifty-eight-year-old professional, had psoriasis for over twenty years. His main symptoms were dry, reddish-purple lesions on his legs, arms, hands, and body. The lesions were itchy whenever they flared up. He was about twenty pounds overweight and drank alcohol regularly. Traditional Chinese medicine diagnosis revealed that his pulse was wiry and irregular, and his tongue was purple.

We suggested that Steve drink more water, that he consider going on the Digestive Clearing Program and try limiting his consumption of wheat-containing foods. We also recommended that he incorporate more fatty fish into his diet. He was asked to take Skin Balance (2 tablets three times a day), Mobility 2 (3 tablets three times a day), and a supplement high in EPA and DHA (3 capsules daily with meals) in order to control the inflammatory response.

After three weeks Steve reported that the lesions were less itchy and red. However, he felt agitated from following the Digestive Clearing Program and from not having alcohol for one week. We noticed that he had smoked a cigarette in the parking lot while waiting for his appointment. When we inquired, he said that for several months he had been trying to cut down to a few cigarettes per day, but that not drinking alcohol was increasing his cigarette cravings. His pulse was more wiry, and his tongue was dry and purple. We suggested he continue the herbs at the same dosage, and increase the EPA/DHA to 6 capsules daily with meals. We also referred him to an acupuncturist to help ease the cigarette cravings and to treat the neck pain he was also experiencing.

Steve returned in three weeks showing considerable improvement. The skin lesions were starting to shrink; they were mostly pink instead of reddish-purple, and were less itchy. His pulse was less wiry than his previous visits, but his tongue was unchanged. The acupuncture treatments helped him cut down to one cigarette a day, and reduced his neck pain. He abandoned the Digestive Clearing Program after two weeks, but noticed a correlation between alcohol and wheat consumption and the itching. Although Steve was willing to eliminate bread from his diet, he did not want to eliminate alcohol entirely. We recommended that he continue on the Skin Balance (2 tablets four times a day) and Mobility 2 (3 tablets four times a day), and EPA/DHA (6 capsules per day).

After two months, all Steve's symptoms were improving, so we adjusted his herbal protocol to Skin Balance (2 tablets four times a day). Mobility 2 was stopped and Marrow Plus (2 tablets four times a day) was added to build his blood. The EPA/DHA dosage remained the same. He continued taking the herbs for six months with total resolution of the psoriasis.

Discussion: Steve's tongue and lesions were purplish, indicating blood stasis, while his being overweight and the presence of a lingering condition, i.e., the psoriasis, indicated dampness. The formula Skin Balance was used to clear the liver: in the biomedical model, alcohol is toxic to the liver, and in the Chinese model, alcohol is too warming to both the liver and to the body in general. Although Steve was reluctant to eliminate alcohol totally, he was able to reduce his consumption to one to two drinks on the weekends only. This helped keep the psoriasis under control.

The formula Mobility 2 was used to increase blood circulation and drain dampness, and Marrow Plus was selected to help tonify the blood in order to relieve itching. A six-month course of treatment is not unusual for stubborn cases of psoriasis.

Case #2

Edwina, a forty-two-year-old musician, suffered from psoriasis for thirty-seven years. The lesions affected her entire body and were especially severe on her arms and legs, where the plaques were purple, thick, and scaly. During flare-ups, her skin was very itchy, particularly at night. Flare-ups were treated with ultraviolet radiation and the corticosteroid, triamcinolone. She was aware that corn, chocolate, fruit, wheat, and peanuts made her symptoms worse. She also complained of poor digestion and abdominal pain, and occasional hot flashes, as she was perimenopausal. Edwina led a hectic life—teaching during the day, performing in the evenings, in addition to traveling to performances. Thus, it was no surprise that when she came to our clinic she indicated that for over a year she had been experiencing fatigue with difficulty rising in the morning. Traditional Chinese medicine diagnosis revealed that her pulse was weak and slow, and her tongue was pink, dry, and cracked, with a yellow coating.

After evaluating her overall situation, in particular her diet, we recommended that Edwina eat more lean meat and salmon, as she was consuming a preponderance of carbohydrates. When she was on the road, she usually ate things that triggered flare-ups of her psoriasis. We also urged her to chew her food carefully, as she was prone to eating quickly. She was also asked to take the formulas Colostroplex (1 tablet per day), Skin Balance (2 tablets three times a day), and Quiet Digestion (1 to 2 tablets three times a day). She was instructed to start with 2 tablets of Skin Balance three times a day, but to reduce to 1 three times a day if she developed loose stools.

After two weeks Edwina reported her skin was much less itchy; however, she complained of stomach pain. Her pulse was wiry, slightly irregular, and weak in the first and third positions. Her tongue was still dry, pink, and cracked, with a slightly yellow coating. We recommended she continue with the herbal protocol. To address the stomach pain, we suggested she not eat so much during her evening meal, since she was making up for the day's hunger during this meal. Two weeks later, the lesions on her legs had totally disappeared, and she reported that the itching had improved ninety percent. With past flare-ups, this degree of improvement had usually been attained only with triamcinolone and ultraviolet radiation. This time, by adding the herbal protocol, she required only triamcinolone and many fewer UV treatments.

At this point she reported that bleeding hemorrhoids were her principal complaint, something that she had not indicated when she first came to the clinic. Sometimes she had to get up as many as ten times a night with the urge to defecate. Her pulse was still weak and slow, and her tongue was now pale with a dry, gray coating. We urged her to undergo standard biomedical tests to rule out other possible causes of blood in the stool. We also suggested she reduce Skin Balance (to 1 tablet three times a day), increase Colostroplex (to 4 tablets per day), increase Quiet Digestion (to 3 tablets three times a day), and add Formula H (3 tablets three times a day), a formula specific for hemorrhoids.

Three weeks later, the psoriasis was totally eliminated. During this time, Edwina had decided to go on a three-day vegetable broth fast, which had greatly help reduce her hemorrhoid symptoms. But now she was constipated. The medical tests to determine the cause of blood in the stool were inconclusive. Her pulse was now thin and her tongue was still pale and dry. At this time, Edwina discontinued treatment, as her psoriasis was in remission.

Discussion: As is typical of many persons with psoriasis, Edwina's flare-ups were tied to emotional stress and a poor diet, although in her case, it appeared that her diet was the more significant factor in the flare-ups. As an example, she used chocolate as an instant energy boost, particularly when she was traveling. But she would end up paying for it a few days later by experiencing a flare-up. Once her diet was under control, the skin lesions began healing, and the flare-ups decreased in frequency and severity. Using herbal formulas such as Quiet Digestion helped make the foods she was sensitive to more tolerable. Skin Balance was used not only to heal her skin, but also to promote regular bowel movements so that toxins were eliminated through the stools instead of the skin.

Case #3

Steve, a fifty-year-old landscaper, complained of psoriasis that was characterized by red, itchy lesions on the arms, legs, scalp, and nails. The skin on his face, arms, and hands was particularly rough, probably due to the fact that he worked almost exclusively outdoors in a very windy climate. His diet consisted mainly of fast foods and fried foods, as well as soda. He also drank alcohol regularly. He had tried various medications, but was reluctant to use the methotrexate recommended by his doctor. Traditional Chinese medicine diagnosis revealed that his pulse was slightly slow, and his tongue was pale and dry.

Since Steve's diet was so poor, we suggested he reduce or eliminate his consumption of fast foods and fried foods. We also urged him to eliminate soda and alcohol, and drink at least 64 oz of water daily. We recommended the formula Resinall K (1 part) diluted in safflower oil (3 parts) to be applied twice daily to his arms, legs, and scalp. He was also asked to use Skin Balance (2 tablets four times a day) and Marrow Plus (2 tablets four times a day). One month later, Steve reported that the itching had decreased by fifty percent and that the lesions had shrunk in size by three quarters. Visually his skin looked less red, though his pulse and tongue were unchanged. We reduced Skin Balance (to 1 tablet four times a day) and increased Marrow Plus (to 3 tablets four times a day). After three months on this protocol, the lesions were gone and Steve reported that his itching had improved by ninety percent. He continued to take Marrow Plus (3 tablets, 3 to 4 times daily) for another six months, and used the topical formula as needed. He also reported that his diet was much healthier—he was eating more vegetables and fruits, and drinking plenty of water.

Case #4 Psoriatic Arthritis

Grace, a fifty-six-year-old manager, had a twelve-year history of psoriasis. In addition, for several years she had been struggling with arthritis and temperomandibular joint (TMJ) syndrome. The psoriasis was present on her knuckles, elbows, knees, toes, and head. The lesions were purple, thick, and scaly, and itched during flare-ups. Her hands were especially affected by both the arthritis and psoriasis. She had tried numerous topical and internal pharmaceutical treatments, including methoxtrexate injections. Traditional Chinese medicine diagnosis revealed that her pulse was wiry and her tongue was reddish-purple.

We recommended Quercenol, an antioxidant formula, and fish oil capsules (2 capsules three times a day with meals), along with Mobility 2 (3 tablets three times a day between meals) and Skin Balance (1 tablet three times a day between meals). We also suggested she eat cold-water fish such as salmon, mackerel, and tuna, which contain high levels of omega-3 oils, which help reduce inflammation. After three weeks, Grace noticed a slight decrease in the joint pain and swelling as well as in the itching, though her pulse and tongue were unchanged. We recommended she continue with the protocol, but increase the dosage of Skin Balance (to 3 tablets three times a day), and apply Resinall K topically to the skin lesions (3 times daily).

After one month Grace noticed a major improvement in symptoms. She reported a fifty percent reduction in pain, and substantial improvement in the lesions and itching. Grace remained on the protocol for several more months, with almost complete elimination of her symptoms. Subsequently she elected to stop the herbs, but to continue taking the antioxidant formula and fish oil capsules, and eat fish several times per week.

Rosacea

Rosacea is chronic inflammation of the skin on the cheeks and nose. It is characterized by flushing of the skin, and may also cause a red bulb-like nose, known as rhinophyma, or the "W. C. Fields nose." Acne-like lesions are sometimes present. Rosacea is most common in fair-skinned women between the ages of thirty and fifty. The biomedical cause is not known. The mite *Demodex folliculorum* has been implicated, but as a cause, remains unproven. Standard biomedical treatments include antibiotics and laser therapy. Identifying triggers that bring on flushing and blushing is often helpful in decreasing the severity of the condition. Such triggers may include alcohol and spicy foods, sunlight, heat, and embarrassment. It may be helpful to further eliminate dairy, fried foods, iodized salt, and sweets, since these can give rise to internal heat, which can lead to facial flushing.

Self-Treatments

- Vinegar (1 tsp in water, taken with meals): To aid digestion.
- High-potency antioxidant with zinc.
- Vitamin A (up to 50,000 IU daily) until skin clears. Vitamin A should be used cautiously during pregnancy; consult your healthcare professional about dosages over 5,000 IU.
- Acidophilus/bifidus: This product supports naturally present, beneficial bacteria in the body, which eventually will eliminate pathogenic bacteria (follow label directions).

Professional Treatments

- ◆ To nourish fluids, add Nine Flavor Tea (3 tablets three times a day) to tonify yin, or Great Yin (3 tablets three times a day) to tonify yin and clear heat.
  - ■ To further clear heat, add Coptis Purge Fire (1 to 3 tablets three times a day).
- ◆ Coptis Purge Fire wash: Crush 2 tablets, simmer in 32 oz water for 5 minutes, then steep for 15 minutes. Apply to affected area with washcloth 1 to 2 times daily.

Case Studies

Case #1

Clare, a forty-year-old office manager, had rosacea that covered most of her face. She had the condition for over a year. Her doctor had prescribed long-term antibiotics and recommended she use sunscreen when outdoors. He also counseled her to avoid alcohol and spicy foods. Traditional Chinese medicine diagnosis revealed that her pulse was sinking and slightly fast, and her tongue was red with a moist yellow coating.

As Clare had been on antibiotics continuously for three months, and she presented with signs of damp-heat, we felt strongly that she was experiencing some kind of yeast infection. We therefore suggested Phellostatin (2 tablets four times a day) for its antifungal properties. To help resolve the damp-heat as indicated by the moist yellow tongue coating, we recommended she reduce or eliminate dairy products, sweets, and all sodas. Clare's pulse revealed yin deficiency, so we suggested Nine Flavor Tea (3 tablets four times a day). We also advised her to counter her cravings for sweets with fresh fruits, and to increase her intake of fresh vegetables and lean protein. She was asked to take the herbs with peppermint tea since it is cooling in nature.

After two weeks there was a noticeable improvement in Clare's rosacea. Her tongue was red, but no longer had the moist yellow coating; her pulse was unchanged. Because the rosacea had improved so much, we encouraged her to consult her physician about reducing or discontinuing the antibiotics, which he agreed to. After staying on the protocol for two more months, Clare's rosacea resolved completely.

Case #2

Rick, a twenty-nine-year-old cook, complained of rosacea around the nose. He also had dry, itchy skin, and burning eyes. All of these symptoms were aggravated by his job, which required him to spend a great deal of time around ovens and gas burners. His face was flushed and felt hot. He also had bleeding gums. Traditional Chinese medicine diagnosis revealed that his tongue was red with a thick yellow coating, and his pulse was slightly rapid.

We recommended the formulas Coptis Purge Fire (2 tablets four times a day) and Nine Flavor Tea (2 tablets four times a day) to reduce heat and nourish yin. We also suggested Rick apply a Coptis Purge Fire wash to the area affected by rosacea twice per day. He was counseled about reducing or eliminating alcohol, sweets, spicy foods, dairy products, fruit juice, and shellfish, and to increase his consumption of fresh vegetables and water.

After two weeks there was a slight improvement in all symptoms, so we encouraged Rick to remain on the protocol. After four weeks he reported an eighty to ninety percent improvement in all symptoms. His pulse was normal. His tongue was still red, but the thick yellow coating now covered only the back of his tongue. As he became more aware of his diet, he had noticed that his skin symptoms were aggravated by alcohol and chocolate, so he immediately stopped consuming them. We suggested he reduce the Coptis Purge Fire (to 1 tablet four times a day), and continue taking Nine Flavor Tea (2 tablets four times a day). Rick was encouraged to adhere to the diet as much as possible, and to apply the Coptis Purge Fire wash if the rosacea recurred.

Two months later Rick's skin had cleared. He reduced his hours as a cook and was looking for new work. He was also emotionally more upbeat.

Case #3

Rob, a thirty-six-year-old office worker, presented with acne rosacea. He also complained of tiredness, abdominal cramping and intestinal gas, as well as constipation, which sometimes alternated with diarrhea. He was fifty to sixty pounds overweight. He frequently felt hot, and his face was very red, especially the cheeks. Traditional Chinese medicine diagnosis revealed that his pulse was slippery, and his tongue red and dry.

We recommended Rob take Quiet Digestion (2 tablets with each meal) and Clearing (3 tablets two times a day). We also suggested that he reduce or eliminate dairy products, alcohol, fried and fatty foods, sweets, and coffee from his diet, since these promote heat in the body. He was also asked to increase his intake of non-gas producing vegetables, and to eat protein with every meal. The increase in protein was aimed at addressing his tiredness. Though we would have given him herbs that would more strongly nourish yin, we used Clearing because we were concerned that the rich yin tonics in classic formulas such as Rehmannia 6 or Nine Flavor Tea would make his digestive symptoms worse. Quiet Digestion was administered to help Rob digest his food and eliminate cramping and reduce gas.

Three weeks later, Rob reported significant improvements in his digestive symptoms and his energy level. His face was less flushed, but he was still constipated. We recommended that he continue taking Clearing and Quiet Digestion at the same dosages. He was also asked to take a teaspoon of freshly ground flaxseeds with a large glass of water everyday, and that he use flaxseed oil as a salad dressing. Rob's herbal protocol was altered over time in response to the positive changes he experienced; gradually his rosacea and digestive symptoms improved, and he was able to lose weight.

Note: Flaxseeds and flax oil contain essential fatty acids, which not only help alleviate constipation but also have anti-inflammatory properties which may help reduce rosacea symptoms.

Sarcoidosis

Sarcoidosis is an autoimmune disease that causes inflammation throughout the body. Many organ systems are involved, with the lungs, liver, spleen, lymph nodes, and eyes being most frequently affected. The skin is involved in twenty to twenty-five percent of cases. Skin symptoms can include bluish-purple areas on the face, and red bumps on the legs. Generalized symptoms include joint and muscle pain, fatigue, fever, lung problems, swollen lymph nodes, blurred vision, dry eyes, aversion to light, and weight loss. Biomedical treatment uses steroids to reduce inflammation.

Self-Treatments

- Antioxidant formula (follow label directions).
- Power Mushrooms (2 tablets three times a day) for fatigue. Reduce or discontinue using if you feel unusually warm.
- Seaweed may help to address lymph node swelling (eat several times a week).

Professional Treatments

- Astra Isatis (3 tablets three times a day): Use to boost the immune system and detoxify lymph.
  - For dry eyes and other signs of heat, add Nine Flavor Tea (3 tablets three times a day).
  - For inflammation, add Resinall E (3 tablets three times a day).
  - For fatigue and signs of cold add Power Mushrooms (1 to 2 tablets three times a day).
- Mobility 2 and Clear Heat (2 tablets each four times a day): Use for joint pain accompanied by fever.
- Resinall K: Apply topically to lesions full strength, or dilute 1 part Resinall K in 3 parts hot water or 3 parts vegetable oil.
- Thymus extract (follow label directions).

Scabies

Scabies is a skin infestation caused by a type of mite that burrows into the skin to lay eggs. Symptoms of scabies include small, gray, scaly swellings, often located between the fingers, on the wrists and genitals, and in the armpits. In later stages of infestation there may be reddish lumps on the limbs or trunk. Intense itching, especially at night, is considered the hallmark of this condition. Scabies is usually spread through direct physical contact with an infected person, or with their personal items such as clothing, towels, or sheets. Standard biomedical treatment is to apply scabicides such as Lindane, sulfur, permethrin, or crotamiton topically over the entire body from the neck down. Lindane is banned in California, as it is a nerve toxin leading to many side effects. Shampoos and creams with Lindane when rinsed off pollute the water supply. All family members and sexual partners should be treated. Intimate articles of clothing, bed linen, and towels should be soaked in bleach, and washed and dried using the hot cycle. Natural treatments may be used in conjunction with these treatments, or if the above medications do not work.

Self-Treatments

- Bergamot oil: Mix 5 drops per 1 tsp hot water (increase amounts proportionally if more is needed). Let cool and apply head to toe, 2 to 3 times daily.
- Thyme, peppermint, lavender remedy: Mix 5 drops of each essential oil per 2 tbsp vegetable oil (increase amounts proportionally if more is needed). Apply head to toe 2 to 3 times daily.

Professional Treatments

- Chaparral wash: Simmer 1 tsp chaparral for 5 minutes per 8 oz water, then steep for 15 minutes. Apply with a washcloth 2 to 3 times per day, covering the entire body from head to toe. Several drops of bergamot oil may be added to the wash to increase its efficacy if chaparral alone is not effective after two days of use.
- Cir-Q wash: Grind 2 to 4 tablets, mix with 8 oz of boiling water and let steep for 2 hours, stirring occasionally. Apply with a washcloth 3 times daily. Hot water can be added several more times; initial liquid can be used over two- to three-day period. If results are not seen in three days, add equal parts 3 drops Resinall K to the Cir-Q wash.
- Resinall K: Dilute 1 part Resinall K in 3 parts hot water. Apply 2 to 3 times daily.

Case Study

Ron, a twenty-eight-year-old salesman, contracted scabies from his girlfriend who worked in a hospital. He had tried three different medications (Lindane, benzyl benzoate, and permethrin), had seen two different dermatologists, and was diligent about his personal hygiene. Despite these measures the scabies persisted. Traditional Chinese medicine diagnosis revealed that his pulse was slow and sinking, and his tongue was reddish-purple.

We recommended crushing 4 Cir-Q tablets, mixing this with 8 ounces of boiling water, steeping for 2 hours, and applying with a washcloth twice daily from head to toe, including the face and scalp. After two weeks the condition had resolved completely.

Discussion: This formula has worked for several clients with drug-resistant scabies. Both Cir-Q and Resinall K contain natural insecticides. One case that was successfully resolved involved alternately applying Cir-Q and Resinall K. The Resinall K was mixed with rubbing alcohol (1 part to 4 parts) and applied to the entire surface of the skin, including the face and scalp. Another successfully resolved case of drug-resistant scabies involved alternately applying Cir-Q and Resinall K for two weeks, followed by one week of chaparral washes.

Scaling (Ichthyosis)

Ichthyosis is called the "fish scale disease" to explain the dry scaly skin. It is an inherited disease which usually first occurs in childhood. It may disappear for years and then return. Typically, it is found on the elbows, knees, hands, and may worsen in the winter. Petroleum jelly (Vaseline) may be applied to affected areas. For best results, apply Vaseline to troubled areas and wrap these areas in plastic before going to bed. Cold creams and lactic acid containing lotions should be applied twice or more each day.

Self-Treatments

- Vitamin E (400 to 800 IU per daily).
- Vitamin A (10,000 to 50,000 IU daily). Do not take more than 5,000 IU during pregnancy.
- Flax (1 to 3 tbsp daily of fresh ground seeds or flaxseed oil).
- Fish oil containing EPA/DHA (3 to 10 g per day or 1 to 3 tsp of cod liver oil daily).

Professional Treatments

- Skin Balance (2 to 3 tablets three to four times a day). For red, itchy skin, add Clear Heat (1 to 3 tablets three to four times a day): for stronger results, add Marrow Plus (2 to 3 tablets three to four times a day) for blood deficiency.
- For yin deficiency, use Nine Flavor Tea (3 tablets three times a day) plus Coptis Purge Fire (1 to 3 tablets three times a day).
- Spring Wind Ointment (use as directed, 2 to 3 times a day).
- Resinall K: Mix 1 part Resinall K to 3 parts safflower oil and apply topically 2 to 3 times a day.

Scleroderma

Scleroderma means "hard skin." In addition to a thickening and tightening of the skin, there may be joint pain and stiffness, and swelling of the hands and feet in the morning. It is thought that scleroderma is either an autoimmune disease or a blood vessel defect that causes excessive collagen build up. Raynaud's phenomenon, a condition where the skin of the fingers turns from white to blue to pinkish, following cold exposure or stress, is common in scleroderma patients. In some cases, hypertension, kidney failure, lung complications, and intestinal problems are also seen. Exercise is often recommended to help reduce stiffness and to improve blood flow. It is also recommended that you quit smoking, and that you keep your body, especially your hands and feet, warm at all times. Medications depend on the signs and symptoms. For example, blood dilators are used if Raynaud's is present, analgesics are used for pain, and drugs may be used to reduce blood pressure.

Self-Treatments

- Fish oil containing EPA/DHA (3 to 10 g a day or cod liver oil 1 to 3 tsp a day). Flax (use 1 to 3 tbsp of freshly ground flaxseeds or flax oil).
- Broad-spectrum antioxidant (use as directed).
- Gotu Kola (1,000 to 4,000 mg daily).

Professional Treatments

- Mobility 2 and Flavonex (2 tablets of each formula four times a day) to reduce stiffness and improve blood flow.
- Resinall K: Mix 1 part Resinall K with 3 parts safflower oil and apply topically 2 to 3 times a day.
- If in cold condition, add hot ginger compress: add powdered ginger to boiling water for five minutes, steep ten minutes, apply to handcloth, then massage into skin.

Sebaceous Cysts

Sebaceous cysts are growths containing protein and sebum (oil from the skin). Typically they appear on the face, scalp, or back; a whitehead is a small sebaceous cyst. These cysts are harmless unless they become infected. Redness, swelling, and pain characterize infection. In the event of an infection, see your health professional, as antibiotics may be necessary. Eliminating caffeine, dairy products, fatty and fried foods, sweets, and chocolate may help prevent sebaceous cysts from forming.

Self-Treatments

- Black currant oil (six 500 mg capsules per day) or flaxseed, ground fresh, and flax oil (1 to 3 tbsp per day).
- Goldenseal tincture can be applied topically.
- Drink burdock tea (do not use if you have loose stools or diarrhea).
- Vitamin A (10,000 to 25,000 IU daily). Consult your doctor if you are pregnant.
- Vitamin E topically. Break open capsule and apply topically.

Professional Treatments

- Coptis Purge Fire: Take 3 tablets three times a day and apply as a wash. Clean area with hydrogen peroxide first. Simmer two tablets in 16 oz of water for 5 minutes and apply to cysts with a cotton swab.
- Bupleurum Entangled Qi (3 tablets three times a day). This is used long-term to increase blood circulation and to reduce the size of the cysts.

Seborrhea (Seborrheic Dermatitis)

Seborrhea is scaling caused by malfunction of the sebaceous (oil secreting) glands. Typically it occurs on the scalp, face, and chest. Seborrheic skin may be greasy or dry and flaky; the scales may form large patches. According to James Balch, M.D., and Phyllis Balch, CNC, seborrhea may be linked to lack of biotin, vitamin A, and other nutrients or a yeast, Pityrosporum orbiculare, which normally lives in the hair follicles.[17] Other factors may be stress, oily skin, obesity, and other skin disorders. Physicians may prescribe sulfur-containing drugs or Diprosone cream. Consider eliminating gluten-containing foods such as wheat, chocolate, dairy products, nuts, shellfish, nuts, and sweets. (See Eczema treatments.) Wear loose-fitting clothing made of natural fibers, such as cotton, that breathe. Over-the-counter shampoos containing zinc may be helpful.

Self-Treatments

- Everclean, Home Health Products shampoo (keep on hair for 30 minutes or overnight) before washing.
- Black currant oil (6 times 500 mg per day) or Flax (1 to 3 tbsp of fresh ground seeds or flax oil) or fish oil supplement (3 to 10 g per day).
- B-complex (50 mg, 1 to 3 times per day) plus 100 mg of PABA.
- Biotin (500 mcg three times per day) with meals.
- Zinc as part of an antioxidant preparation. (Take 50 mg zinc per day.)
- Vitamin E (400 to 800 IU).
- Vitamin A (up to 50,000 IU); do not use more than 5,000 IU during pregnancy.

♦ Cedarwood essential oil, topically (3 drops in 2 tsp of vegetable oil). You may add tea tree oil (3 drops) for stronger effects.

Professional Treatments

♦ Nine Flavor Tea: Take this when symptoms include signs of yin deficiency, including dryness and afternoon fever (3 tablets three times a day).
♦ Marrow Plus: For blood deficiency, dryness, itching, pallor, and fatigue (3 tablets three to four times a day).
♦ Skin Balance (2 to 3 tablets three to four times a day) with itching and redness. Reduce dosage if loose stools are noticed. Skin balance can be combined with the above formulas.

Case Studies

Case #1 Seborrhea

Bob, a forty-eight-year-old gardener, suffered from seborrheic dermatitis, headache, and fatigue. His doctor had prescribed topical steroids. He had a history of ulcerative colitis and swollen lymph nodes. His pulse was rapid and his tongue was reddish-purple. We recommended a combination of Skin Balance (2 tablets three times a day) and Clear Heat (2 tablets three times a day). Because Bob was suffering from excess heat symptoms, we suggested he reduce or eliminate alcohol, caffeine, and spicy food. Bob returned two weeks later and he was disappointed that his condition was essentially the same, although he had a few days where there was less itching. We encouraged him to continue with the herbal protocol, and because he had no loose stools, we suggested he increase this regimen to three of each product three times a day. We asked if he had been able to reduce his beer drinking, caffeine, and spicy food. He said he was trying to eat less Mexican food, but that he was still drinking almost every night, and he was hooked on espresso. We encouraged him to follow through with the dietary recommendations; otherwise he might not be able to get off steroids.

He returned in three weeks. There was significantly less redness, itching, and scaling, and his headaches were reduced. His pulse was less rapid, but his tongue was still reddish-purple. He now complained of dandruff, and so in addition to the herbal protocol he was also asked to use a zinc-based shampoo for his scalp.

He returned a month later with all symptoms ninety percent improved. He said that he found it difficult but had reduced his alcohol, caffeine, and spicy food. He had increased his water intake and was drinking less soda. His pulse was slightly fast and his tongue was still reddish-purple. At this point, we adjusted his protocol to Skin Balance (2 tablets three times a day) and Nine Flavor Tea (3 tablets three times a day). Nine Flavor Tea replaced the Clear Heat, as we felt yin-nourishing and less heat-clearing was required.

Case #2

Paul, a twenty-five-year-old massage therapist, complained of seborrheic dermatitis and indigestion. He had visited an acupuncturist who had told him he was yin deficient and prescribed Rehmannia, which did not help his skin and made his digestion worse. He had also been to several dermatologists and had been prescribed various remedies. His pulse was soggy, and his tongue was red with a yellow coating. We recommended he follow an anti-yeast diet, omitting alcohol, dairy, sweets, and yeast-containing foods such as breads and pastries. We recommended Quiet Digestion to improve his digestive functioning (2 tablets three times a day) and Phellostatin, and an antifungal and antibacterial formula (1 tablet three times a day for the first week, 2 tablets three times a day thereafter). We also recommended Everclean shampoo lathered onto the scalp for thirty minutes before rinsing, every day for a week, five minutes before rinsing, thereafter.

Two weeks later, he told us that his scalp had felt better than it had in years. He felt his skin was less irritated, and his digestion was improved. His pulse was less soggy, and his tongue was normal. He continued taking Phellostatin for two months, and continued to use the Quiet Digestion on an as-needed basis. His skin was ninety percent improved, and he rarely had indigestion. He attributed his results to the herbs and elimination of sweets, bread and pastries, and limiting his alcohol consumption.

Shingles (Herpes Zoster)

Shingles is caused by the same virus that causes chickenpox. The virus can remain dormant in nerve cells for many years after the onset of chickenpox. The first symptom of a herpes zoster attack is usually pain or tingling over the area that is to be affected. A few days later a red rash appears. The red bumps soon turn to virus-filled blisters which then dry, crust, and turn yellow. Eruptions usually occur on only one side of the body, either over the ribs, on one half of the face, or as a strip on one half of the neck and adjoining arm, or on the lower body.

Typically shingles strikes the elderly and those with suppressed immune systems. Postherpetic neuralgia is pain due to nerve damage. It may be serious and persist for many months. A herpes zoster attack accompanied by eye pain should be reported to a physician immediately, as ophthalmic herpes zoster may have serious complications. Standard biomedical treatments for herpes zoster include analgesics for pain, soothing lotions, wet compresses, and steroids. Acyclovir taken at the first sign of an outbreak may lessen the severity of the attack.

Self-Treatments

- Myrrh tincture: Take internally one-half to 1 dropperful (3 to 4 times daily); and apply topically to affected area (3 times daily).
- Antioxidant formula that contains zinc and selenium (follow label instructions).
- St. John's wort oil: Apply topically to affected area (3 to 4 times daily). This is effective for pain in many patients.
- Lemon balm tea: Steep 1 tbsp dried lemon balm leaves in 1 cup boiled water for 15 minutes. Strain and apply as a warm or cool compress depending on preference (3 to 4 times daily). Lemon balm stops viral replication.

Professional Treatments

Chinese herbal therapy includes the administration of tonic herbs to strengthen the immune system, herbal antivirals, and the use of specific pain-relieving herbs used topically as well as internally.

- Astra Isatis (3 tablets three times a day): Use to strengthen the immune system and to clear virus. For fever and areas that feel hot to the touch, add Clear Heat (1 to 3 tablets three times a day). Clear Heat can also be used as a wash (3 to 4 times a day) and as a poultice (change 2 times a day).

- Mobility 2 (3 tablets three to four times a day) is especially useful for pain that migrates. Combine with Clear Heat for heat signs or Astra Isatis if the patient is weak.
- Power Mushrooms (2 to 3 tablets three times a day): Use to boost the immune system. This is especially useful for cold signs when combined with Astra Isatis long-term.
- Resinall K (one-half dropperful three to four times a day taken internally): Massage into affected area several times a day. Can be combined with powdered selenium or Clear Heat to form a poultice, which is applied twice daily. Cover with gauze.
- Channel Flow can be used (2 to 3 tablets three to four times a day) with the above measures to reduce pain.
- Use a moxa stick to warm the painful area for thirty minutes each day for three consecutive days. If the client's skin becomes too warm, temporarily move the moxa stick to LI 4, ST 36, or points along the liver channel, before returning to the affected area. Moxabustion is used to reduce pain and attack virus.

Case Studies

Case #1

Larry, a retired seventy-nine-year-old, had shingles with burning pain affecting the left side of his face and scalp. Because the pain was severe, he was being treated with Ativan, Darvocet, and valproic acid. Larry was referred to our clinic by an acupuncturist who had been able to control the pain for only short periods of time. Larry's pulse was irregular, and his tongue was reddish-purple and dry.

We recommended Clear Heat (2 tablets four times a day) to reduce toxic heat. Resinall K was also suggested to be taken internally (one-half dropperful four times a day), and applied topically twice daily after washing his face with soap and water. After one week, Larry reported slightly less pain, but indicated that he had developed diarrhea, which he believed was caused by the herbs. When we probed Larry, he admitted that the diarrhea could have been caused by some spoiled food he had eaten from a deli. Nevertheless, we added Astra Isatis (2 tablets four times a day) to his protocol, as it contains strengthening herbs that would counter the cooling nature of Clear Heat in case it was in fact the cause of the diarrhea.

After three weeks, Larry came in unhappy about the number of pills he was taking and about the taste of Resinall K; however, he reported being able to cut back on the Darvocet, which helped him feel less drowsy. Over the next couple of months, as his pain and heat signs diminished, the Clear Heat was stopped. He remained on the Resinall K for another two months, and on the Astra Isatis for six months. When we followed up with him at this point, Larry indicated that his pain was much improved.

Case #2

Harold, an eighty-year-old, suffered from shingles following chemotherapy treatments for colon cancer. His pulse was sinking and rapid, and his tongue was scarlet.

We recommended Astra Isatis (3 tablets four times a day), and that he apply Resinall K topically to the affected parts of his body by massaging it into the area twice per day. He was also asked to take Resinall K internally (one-half dropperful four times a day). Within three weeks, Harold obtained substantial pain relief. He continued on the Resinall K for another two weeks before discontinuing it, and continued on the Astra Isatis for another six months. Harold reported no further outbreaks of shingles.

Skin Allergies

Contact dermatitis (skin allergies) is an irritation of the skin caused by plants, cosmetics, chemicals, metals, or drugs. Allergies are a response from the immune system to anything considered foreign. This causes a red, itchy rash to form, followed by swelling and blistering. Some allergic reactions produce a burning sensation in the eyes, mouth, and throat. The most common irritants include poison ivy, poison oak, poison sumac, ragweed, chrysanthemum, oranges, potatoes, nickel (used in jewelry), rubber, preservatives, chemicals used in cosmetics, printing, paint, and leather processing. Irritants may also be found in petroleum, permanent press clothing, dry cleaning, household cleaning agents, foam insulation, particleboard, rugs, agricultural products such as pesticides and herbicides, and food additives.

Reactions are triggered when a sensitive person comes in direct contact (by touching), or indirect contact (coming in contact with clothing or pet fur that has come in contact with the allergen). It is also possible to get a reaction through breathing in allergens (chemicals in the air). A rash can develop immediately after exposure, or it can take up to two days. Obviously, it is best to avoid contact with an allergen in order to prevent a reaction. If you know you have come into contact with an allergen, it is best to wash your skin thoroughly with soap and water. It is important to wash any clothing that has come in contact with an irritant. Over-the-counter creams containing calamine may be applied topically and antihistamines may be taken internally. Plants detoxify work environments to a certain extent. Hang clothes outdoors after dry cleaning. Use natural cleaning products found at health food stores, and use environmental friendly products whenever possible.

186

Self-Treatments

- Make a topical paste with baking soda and water. Take an Epsom salt bath (with essential oils).

Professional Treatments

- Xanthium Relieve Surface (3 tablets three times a day).
- Astra C (1 tablet three times a day) over a long term to reduce allergic response.
- Colostroplex (1 to 4 tablets a day) supports the immune system and reduces the allergic response over time.

Case Study (Poison Oak)

Carol, a thirty-four-year-old female, had extreme facial swelling due to inhaling poison oak that was being burned near where she was camping. She had a previous history of poison oak allergy and wanted to avoid using steroid medication. Her pulse was wiry, and her tongue was normal. We recommended Xanthium Relieve Surface formula (3 tablets six times a day) for a few days. We also suggested she consult with a doctor or pharmacist about using an antihistamine product. She took the herbs along with an oral antihistamine and the swelling was relieved in three days.

Skin Cancer

Skin cancer is one of the most common forms of cancer in the U.S. It is usually curable if detected early. Most skin cancers are due to sun exposure—especially repeated sunburns in childhood—and affect the exposed areas on the face, neck, and arms. The best treatment is prevention, that is, avoiding unnecessary sun exposure. If you need to be out in the sun, apply sunscreen that has a sun protection factor (SPF) of at least 15. Reapply the sunscreen often, especially after swimming or perspiring heavily. Wear sunglasses, a hat, and cover your arms and legs whenever possible. Sunlamps, such as those used in tanning salons, are as dangerous as, if not more than, natural sunlight, and so should be avoided.

The major types of skin cancer are basal cell carcinoma, squamous cell carcinoma, and malignant melanoma. A fourth type, Kaposi's sarcoma, primarily affects individuals infected with the human immunodeficiency virus (HIV). (See "Kaposi's Sarcoma," earlier in the chapter.)

Basal cell carcinoma is the most common form of skin cancer in the U.S. Lesions may vary greatly in appearance, from small shiny papules to ulcerated, crusted lesions. A basal cell carcinoma may also appear as a small wavy bump on the face, ears, or neck, as a darkened or flesh-colored lump on the back or torso, or as an unusual skin blemish that repeatedly crusts or bleeds then heals, only to recur again. Some basal cell carcinomas are difficult to differentiate from psoriasis or dermatitis.

Though most basal cell carcinomas are highly curable, especially if detected early, occasionally a lesion can metastasize and even cause death if it invades underlying vital structures. Biomedical treatments include surgical removal, freezing, or radiation therapy.

Squamous cell carcinomas also vary greatly in appearance from red, scaly, or crusted lesions to nodules that may resemble a wart. Though most likely to occur on an area frequently exposed to sun, they may occur anywhere on the body, including in a burn scar or in a pre-existing actinic keratosis (a hard, gray, or dark lesion). Like basal cell carcinomas, squamous cell carcinomas are highly curable, and are usually removed by surgery or freezing.

The most serious kind of skin cancer is malignant melanoma. Melanoma often develops on sun-exposed areas of the skin, but may occur anywhere on the body. The growth may also develop from a pre-existing mole. Moles or growths with one or more of the following characteristics are suspicious and should be examined by a dermatologist as soon as possible:

- Asymmetry: To determine if a mole or growth is asymmetric draw a line through the center. If the two halves are not equal in shape and size, the lesion is asymmetric and should be checked by a dermatologist.
- Borders that are irregular: If the borders are irregular, notched, scalloped, or indistinct (change or spreading of the color from the edge of the mole into the surrounding skin), the growth is suspicious and should be checked.
- Color variation: Melanoma lesions can contain areas of different colors or shades, including browns, blues, reds, whites, and blacks. Any mole that contains more than one color or shade is suspicious and should be checked.
- Diameter greater than 6 millimeters: Any mole larger than 6 millimeters in diameter (approximately the size of a pencil eraser) is suspicious and should be checked.
- Elevation: Any mole that is raised above the surface of the surrounding skin is suspicious and should be checked.

Other signs that a skin lesion may be melanoma are:

- Size: Any change in size, especially sudden or continuous enlargement, is suspicious.
- Surface texture: Bleeding, oozing, crusting, ulceration, erosion, and scaling in a mole are all suspicious signs.
- Sensation: Any mole that is tender, painful, or itchy is suspicious.

- Surrounding skin: Redness, swelling, or new moles in the skin surrounding a mole are all suspicious signs.
- An open sore that does not heal, or heals but then reopens is suspicious.

Untreated, melanoma often spreads rapidly and results in death. However, the cure rate for early stage lesions is excellent. People in high-risk groups—those with many moles, or with pale skin, blue or green eyes, and blond or red hair—should examine their skin for changes in moles or growths at least three times a year. Areas of the skin that are difficult to see should be checked by a spouse, partner, or friend. Those not in high risk groups should examine their skin once per year.

Melanomas are removed by surgery. Chemotherapy and radiation therapy is used in advanced cases. Interferon and other treatments may also be administered.

Self-Treatments

- Antioxidant formula (follow label instructions).
- Green tea appears to have antioxidant and cancer-protecting qualities, therefore it makes sense to substitute green tea for coffee.

Professional Treatments

Herbal formulas are used to augment standard biomedical approaches such as chemotherapy and radiotherapy. They may help strengthen the immune system, thereby countering some of the most harmful effects of these therapies and potentially preventing recurrences. Herbs or supplements should be used only to complement standard biomedical approaches:

- Regeneration (3 tablets three times a day): Tonifies the qi and blood, improves circulation, and removes toxins.
- Astra Essence (3 tablets, three to four times per day): Good overall tonic that supports the qi, blood, yin, and yang.
- Marrow Plus (3 tablets, three to four times per day): Helps increase red and white blood cell counts.
- Ecliptex (2 to 3 tablets, three to four times per day): Helps detoxify the liver.
- Power Mushrooms (2 to 3 tablets three times a day): Helps boost the immune system. It is often combined with the above formulas.

Case Studies

Case #1

Bob, a sixty-six-year-old retiree, had a skin growth for over ten years, which he never thought to have checked. His new family doctor referred him to a dermatologist to have it examined, and it was found to be a melanoma. In addition to having the growth surgically removed he was being treated with chemotherapy and radiation therapy. He was also receiving interferon treatments three times a week. Bob came to our clinic seeking help for low blood counts, constant flu-like symptoms, exhaustion, and depression. Traditional Chinese medicine diagnosis revealed that his pulse was sinking and rapid, and his tongue was red.

Based on his symptoms and on his pulse and tongue presentations, we believed that Bob had yin deficiency. This presentation is rather common among persons receiving chemotherapy

191

and radiation therapy for cancer. Thus, we recommended yin-nourishing and blood-tonifying herbs for Bob. We started him on Nine Flavor Tea (3 tablets four times a day) and Marrow Plus (3 tablets four times a day). We also suggested the antioxidant formula Quercenol (2 tablets two times a day with meals). He was also encouraged to eat a diet rich in fruits and vegetables.

After three weeks Bob said he felt much better. He continued on the protocol for the three remaining months that he was on the biomedical treatments. He made steady improvement in all symptoms. His red blood cell and white blood cell counts also increased.

Case #2

Dorothy, a sixty-three-year-old word processor, was being treated with chemotherapy and radiation therapy for oral cancer. Her skin was inflamed, dry, and cracked, particularly in the upper part of her body. She was experiencing hot flashes, and considerable pain in her jaw where it had been reconstructed during surgery to remove the cancerous tissue. She was taking Tylenol with codeine, and ibuprofen. Traditional Chinese medicine diagnosis revealed that her pulse was thin and wiry and her tongue was reddish purple and dry.

We recommended Nine Flavor Tea (3 tablets three times a day) to nourish the yin. The formula Coptis Purge Fire was used to reduce heat. We started her on 3 tablets three times a day, taken after radiation treatments to reduce the hot flashes. After three days, the Coptis Purge Fire dosage was reduced (to 1 tablet three times a day). Resinall K (one-half dropperful three times a day) was suggested specifically for oral pain and to calm her spirit.

After two weeks, Dorothy noted remarkable improvement of her symptoms. Her skin was less red, she felt less heat sensation, and the Resinall K helped reduce the pain such that she no longer needed the pain medication. She continued on the herbs for six months throughout the duration of her chemo and radiation treatments.

Case #3

Clarence, a sixty-four-year-old plumber, was undergoing chemotherapy for melanoma. His red and white blood cell counts were below normal. In addition, he suffered from fatigue, mild depression, and frequent urination. Traditional Chinese medicine diagnosis revealed that his pulse was sinking and slightly slow, and his tongue was reddish-purple.

We recommended the formulas Marrow Plus and Astra Essence (2 tablets of each four times a day). Four weeks later, Clarence no longer needed to get up at night to urinate, which improved his sleep and his daytime energy level. His pulse was stronger and his tongue looked less purple. He remained on the protocol for three months, the remaining duration of his chemotherapy treatment, after which his blood work showed red and white blood counts within normal ranges. At this point, in order to consolidate the effects of the herbal protocol, we suggested he continue Astra Essence (3 tablets three times a day) and also start taking Coriolus PS (3 tablets three times a day), a medicinal mushroom formula which may have immune-enhancing and cancer protective effects.

Stretch Marks

Stretch marks (striae) are raised, shiny lines on the skin caused by thinning and loss of elasticity of the dermis, the underlying skin layer. Typically they begin as raised red lines, then turn purple, and eventually white as they flatten and fade. Purple stretch marks may also be sign of Cushing's syndrome, a potentially serious hormonal disorder requiring medical treatment. Stretch marks usually develop on the abdomen, breasts, and thighs and are common in pregnant women, weightlifters, and anyone who has had significant weight gain. Retin-A may fade stretch marks if they are recent, however Retin-A is contraindicated for pregnant women. In some cases, experimental laser treatments are used.

Self-Treatments

♦ Massage stretch marks (3 to 4 times daily) with a mixture of 18 drops of essential oil to 3 tablespoons of carrier oil. Essential oils can include myrrh, frankincense, or lavender. Carrier oils can include almond, safflower, or vitamin E oil.

Professional Treatment

♦ Resinall K: Massage stretch marks (3 to 4 times daily) to speed the healing response.

Sunburn

Sunburn is due to damage from the sun's ultraviolet (UV) rays. The most hazardous hours for sun exposure are from 10 am to 2 PM. If you must go out in the sun, use a sunscreen with a sun protection factor (SPF) of at least 15. Wear a hat, and cover as much of your body as possible. Reapply sunscreen after swimming or perspiring heavily. Avoid using perfume or aftershave lotion since these may produce skin discoloration when exposed to sunlight.

It is important to realize that clouds and fog do not block UV radiation, and that UV rays reflected from snow, sand, and water can also burn your skin. Therefore, it is important to protect your skin whenever you are outdoors, even on cloudy winter days. Ultraviolet radiation is more severe at high elevations, so extra protection should be used in mountainous regions. Persons most susceptible to sunburn are those with light skin, blue or green eyes, and blond or red hair. Recurrent sunburn can lead to skin discoloration, actinic keratosis, and most seriously, skin cancer.

Standard biomedical treatments for sunburn include calamine lotion, over-the-counter cortisone creams, aspirin, and in severe cases oral steroids. If your skin blisters after a sunburn, do not break the blisters; rather let them open naturally, then disinfect and cover them.

Self-Treatments

◆ Antioxidant creams that contain vitamin C or green tea may be helpful (follow label directions) to prevent and treat sunburn.

◆ Aloe vera gel or lotion: Apply topically (follow label directions). You may add essential oil for increased effects.

◆ Lemon essential oil: Mix 5 drops per 1 tbsp carrier oil. Apply 3 to 4 times daily.

◆ Lavender essential oil: Mix 5 drops of lavender per 1 tsp carrier oil. Apply 3 to 4 times daily.

◆ Honey may be applied topically several times per day. Honey is not recommended for infants.

◆ Vinegar can be applied topically to reduce burning.

◆ Pineapple: Squeeze juice from two-inch slices of fresh pineapple onto affected areas. Then apply the slices to the affected area for 15 to 20 minutes. This remedy may be used in addition to the above suggestions.

Professional Treatments

- Astra C (2 to 3 tablets three times a day for 1 to 3 weeks). This herbal formula is used in China to speed burn healing.
- Clear Heat wash: Crush 2 tablets and boil in 8 oz water for 5 minutes. Let cool. Apply with a washcloth 3 to 4 times daily.
- Resinall K: Mix 1 part Resinall K with 3 parts water. Apply 3 to 4 times daily.

Case Study

James, a twenty-four-year-old technician, had a severe sunburn with blistering and welts, particularly on his back. Topical aloe vera had not provided any relief. Traditional Chinese medicine diagnosis revealed that his pulse was wiry, and his tongue was red.

We recommended a combination of topical Resinall K and Astra C (2 to 3 tablets three times a day). Resinall K (one-half dropperful) was mixed with 1 tsp water and massaged into the affected skin. After a few days, the sunburn had completely resolved.

Discussion: Astra C contains the traditional formula Jade Screen Powder, which has been used as a Chinese treatment for burns, and zinc to promote healing of the skin.

Sweating Problems

Sweating is the process by which the body vents excessive heat, thereby maintaining the optimal internal temperature to support bodily functions. Sweating for this purpose is usually heaviest on the forehead, upper lip, neck, and chest. Sweating can also be a nervous response, in which case it occurs most heavily on the palms, soles, and armpits.

Excessive sweating, either during the day or at night, that is not induced by exercise, may be a sign of a serious illness such as pneumonia, tuberculosis, tetanus, AIDS, certain types of cancer, malaria, and other diseases.

If you have excessive perspiration that is not induced by exercise, seek a thorough medical diagnosis. If there is no underlying condition, one standard biomedical treatment is aluminum chloride, an ingredient in antiperspirants. Caution using this product may be warranted as there may be a link between excessive intake of aluminum and Alzheimer's disease.

If you do not sweat even during exercise you may lack sweat glands. If so, avoid hot environments, as excessive heat with no adequate venting mechanism can lead to serious conditions such as heat exhaustion or life-threatening heat stroke. You should also have a medical exam to check whether you do in fact lack sweat glands.

Professional Treatments

- Nine Flavor Tea (3 tablets three times a day): Use for excessive sweating due to yin deficiency. Results usually apparent after 3 to 4 weeks' use.
- Tremella and American Ginseng (3 tablets four times a day): Use for severe night sweats with fever.

◆ Shen Gem (3 tablets three to four times a day): Use for excessive sweating day or night due to qi deficiency with pale complexion and slow pulse. Add Astra C (2 tablets three times a day) for strongest effects.

Tinea

Tinea (ringworm) is a group of common fungal infections of the skin. It is caused by a group of fungi called dermatophytes, and can affect the skin, hair, and nails. The common name for tinea is ringworm. Athlete's foot (see earlier section) and jock itch (see earlier section) are forms of tinea. The visible characteristics of tinea vary according to their location. On the body, ringworm manifests as itchy circular patches with a prominent edge, while on the scalp it causes one to several itchy round patches of hair loss. Whitish spots on the shoulders and chest that are resistant to tanning are often tinea versicolor. During the winter, tinea spots can turn darker. This fungal infection is caused by direct or indirect contact. It can also be spread by shared towels and clothing. Some people have a natural resistance to tinea. Tinea infections are spread via contact with other people or animals, or with objects such as chairs, shower stalls, and carpeting.

Biomedical treatment involves topical medications such as selenium sulfide, propylene glycol, or antifungal medications such as griseofulvin (Fulvicin), ketoconazol (Nizoral), terbinafine (Lamisil), and itraconazole (Sporonox). Because these antifungal drugs can be harmful to the liver you may want to explore other treatments before trying them.

Self-Treatments

Mild cases may respond to tea tree oil applied topically. However, one would have to be diligent at applying this remedy, and some people don't like the smell. Typically, it is applied at night before going to bed. Citrus seed oil or oregano essential oil can also be applied. It may take several months to see dramatic results. Herbalists recommend an antifungal diet and supplement program (see "Antifungal Herbs" section) in order to prevent these fungal infections.

Professional Treatments

- Biocidin: Internally: Follow label directions. Topically: Apply directly to affected areas. If irritation occurs, dilute equal parts with water or rubbing alcohol.
- Phellostain (2 to 3 tablets three times a day) for systemic fungus, used for 3 months.

Case Study

Mark is a twenty-four-year-old student who had a recurrent fungal condition diagnosed as tinea versicolor by a dermatologist. In the past he had been prescribed Nizoral, to be taken topically and internally, which usually eradicated the condition; however, it usually came back a few months after treatment. He consulted with us to see if he could avoid using such strong drugs. He also suffered from athlete's foot, alternating diarrhea and constipation (he was diagnosed as having irritable bowel syndrome), and occasional acne outbreaks. He was robust and athletic. His pulse was wiry and slightly rapid and his tongue had a thick gray and yellow coating. We suggested he incorporate the Digestive Clearing Program, and suggested he apply the antifungal herb, oregano, to the fungal rash starting to develop. We also suggested Phellostatin (3 tablets three times a day), which has antifungal properties, and Shu Gan (1 tablet three times a day), a liver-regulating formula, to help his digestion.

He continued with the Phellostatin and Shu Gan for the next six months, applying tea tree oil topically as needed. He no longer had digestive symptoms, and his fungal outbreaks were less frequent and less severe (covered less surface), although he still had to use Nizoral topically. He was able to reduce the dosage and no longer needed oral dosages.

Varicose Veins and Spider Veins

Varicose veins are distended veins just below the surface of the skin. They occur most often on the legs, and may appear blue, purple, swollen, twisted, kinked, or knotted. Varicose veins may cause local itching or pain, and may be accompanied by swelling of the feet and ankles.

It is thought that excess body weight, lack of exercise, and excessive standing contribute to the development of varicose veins. Therefore, regular exercise and slimming down, or maintaining a healthy body weight are important in preventing and resolving this condition. If you have varicose veins and must stand for long periods, elevate your legs above hip level for at least one hour each day, either while on breaks or after work. Elastic support stockings and elevating the foot of your bed two to four inches may also be helpful. Standard biomedical treatments include sclerotherapy (the injection of chemicals into the affected veins), light therapy, and laser surgery.

One particular type of varicose veins is known as idiopathic telangiectases or "spider veins." These are webs of small abnormal veins. Though usually asymptomatic, they can be associated with burning or pain. If extensive they may be considered cosmetically undesirable. Standard biomedical treatment for spider veins is injection of a chemical substance into the local capillaries.

Self-Treatments

+ Cypress oil: Massage the legs (especially the affected areas) once or twice a day with a mixture of 2 drops cypress oil to 1 cup of witch hazel or safflower oil.
+ Horse chestnut: Clinical studies have shown that horse chestnut can help eliminate spider veins by improving circulation and strengthening capillaries and veins. Horse chestnut tablets standardized to contain 50 mg of aescin may be taken twice per day and should be used in conjunction with topical gels containing two percent aescin. Results are usually apparent in three months. Horse chestnut cream may also be applied topically. Use as directed.

Professional Treatments

+ Formula V contains horse chestnut seed extract with synergistic herbs for varicose veins (1 to 2 tablets three times a day). Take for several months.
+ Marrow Plus and Channel Flow (2 tablets of each formula four times a day): Use for qi and blood stagnation characterized by knotted veins and poor circulation.

- Resinall K: Mix 1 part Resinall K with 3 parts witch hazel or safflower oil. Massage into affected area 3 to 4 times daily. This speeds the healing response.
- Mobility 2 and Marrow Plus (2 tablets of each formula four times a day): Use for dampness and poor circulation characterized by a heavy feeling in the legs, fatigue, itching, and purple veins.
- Mobility 2 and Drain Dampness (2 tablets of each formula four times a day): Use for varicose veins accompanied by edema.

Case Studies

Case #1

Mary, a fifty-eight-year-old cashier, complained of varicose veins. She was sixty pounds overweight and had smoked cigarettes intermittently for forty years. She also had hypertension, high cholesterol, and experienced shortness of breath upon exertion. Skin ulcers were apparent above one ankle. Mary was taking blood pressure medication. Traditional Chinese medicine diagnosis revealed that her pulse was slow and irregular, and her tongue was pale with a gray coating.

We recommended Astra Garlic (2 tablets four times a day) to boost qi, reduce cholesterol, and improve cardiovascular function. The formula Channel Flow (2 tablets four times a day) was added to strongly invigorate the blood. We encouraged her to reduce her intake of junk food, and to increase her intake of water, fruit, and vegetables. We particularly recommended grapes, as they appear to improve circulation and capillary health. She was also reminded to elevate her feet during breaks and after work. We gave her AC-Q to use as a nightly foot soak. This was prepared by crushing 1 tablet AC-Q and simmering in 8 oz water for 5 minutes, then combining it with 1 quart warm water in a basin, and soaking the feet for 20 minutes.

Three weeks after we first saw her, Mary reported that she felt about the same. She complained about the number of herbal pills she was having to take, and said that she had not used the foot soak. Her pulse and tongue were unchanged. She agreed to try the herbs in tea form rather than tablets, and promised to start soaking her feet. After two weeks, Mary called to say that she was unable to stomach the tea, and wanted to resume the tablets.

One month after resuming the tablets, Mary said that her varicose veins were improving. She reported a ten percent drop in her cholesterol (her LDL was 263 and now it was 240), and noted that her sleep had also improved. She was taking the recommended dosages of herbs and was soaking her feet 3 times a week. She also reported that she had begun snacking on grapes, which help support capillary integrity, rather than potato chips. Her pulse was also improved in that it was not as slow, but it was still slightly irregular. Her tongue coating was no longer as gray.

Mary remained on the protocol for three more months. At the end of this time, although she had reduced the dosage of herbs on her own (by not coming in for refills), the ulcers above her ankle had healed, and the varicose veins had shrunk in size and were no longer as discolored. She had also lost fifteen pounds. Encouraged by these results, Mary decided to stay on the herbs for another year. Over this period, she continued to lose weight and her varicose veins began disappearing to the point that they were barely noticeable. Her cholesterol was reduced to a normal level.

Case #2

Sandy, a twenty-three-year-old cashier, was overweight and had varicose veins and eczema on her upper legs. She felt embarrassed by her condition. Traditional Chinese medicine diagnosis revealed that Sandy's pulse was slippery, and her tongue was purple with a yellow coating.

We first advised that she abstain from wheat and other gluten-containing foods because of their association with eczema. We suggested that during her breaks and while home, she elevate her legs as much as possible. We then recommended the formula Mobility Two (2 tablets four times a day) to increase blood circulation and rid her body of dampness. Flavonex (2 tablets four times a day) was added to increase blood circulation. Sandy followed this protocol for three months and gradually saw an improvement. She was able to lose some weight. The eczema disappeared, and the varicose veins were not so noticeable.

Vitiligo

Vitiligo is a condition characterized by depigmented white patches of skin. Depigmentation occurs most commonly on the hands, face, groin, and skin folds, but may occur anywhere on the body.

Vitiligo is thought to be an autoimmune disorder, and may be associated with diabetes, hyperthyroidism, adrenal insufficiency, or pernicious anemia. Vitiligo is not contagious but can be a major source of stress for those affected by it. Standard biomedical treatments for vitiligo include controlled exposure to ultraviolet light to induce repigmentation; this is used in combination with medications such as psoralen, which increase photosensitivity. However, up to one hundred sessions may be required, and this is without any guarantee of success. Fluorinated steroids and skin bleaching may be recommended if depigmented areas are extensive.

Self-Treatments

◆ Minimize sun exposure to help keep skin evenly pigmented. When outdoors wear a hat, cover your arms and legs, and apply sunscreen with an SPF of at least 15 to any exposed areas. Reapply after swimming, showering, or perspiring heavily.

◆ Antioxidants: Topical application with vitamin C, carotenoids, green tea, and other antioxidants, may also promote repigmentation. Choose a cream that contains such ingredients and use as directed on the label.

Professional Treatments

◆ Marrow Plus (3 tablets three times a day): Use in conjunction with standard biomedical treatments. To be effective it should be taken for six to twelve months.

◆ Folic acid (10 mg daily) plus vitamin B12 (2 mg daily): Take for 3 to 6 months to encourage repigmentation.[18]

◆ Raw ginger: Mash fresh ginger and apply juice to affected areas 3 to 4 times daily.

◆ Tincture of psoralea (*bu gu zhi*) or tincture of mume (*wu mei*): Massage affected areas with either tincture 2 times daily, followed by sunlight exposure. If rash and blistering of skin results, stop application, and after skin heals, resume treatment at more diluted dosage and/or less frequent applications. Psoralea and mume have been found in Chinese studies to be effective in treating vitiligo, with mume having fewer side effects (rash and blistering) than psoralea. Psoralea contains psoralens, which are strong photosensitizers and promote cell differentiation. Mume contains fruit acids and volatile oils, which also promote new cell growth.[19]

Case Study

Maryann, a thirty-year-old waitress, had vitiligo on her arms and hands. She was overweight, and admitted that she had a sweet tooth. Maryann was taking the antidepressant Prozac and undergoing UV treatments for vitiligo. She was also taking an over-the-counter formula with citrin and chromium for weight loss. Traditional Chinese medicine diagnosis revealed that her pulse was slippery, and her tongue was pale with geographic patches of white and gray coating.

We recommended the formula Marrow Plus to nourish and circulate blood (2 tablets three times a day the first week; 3 three times a day thereafter) and Astra Diet Tea to help counter her sweet tooth and improve digestion. Over the next nine months, Maryann remained on Marrow Plus to improve immune system function. She also continued on the Astra Diet Tea for another two months. Additionally, she underwent UV treatments once weekly, and there was a noticeable reduction, though not total elimination of, the vitiligo.

Warts

Warts are bumps on the skin caused by human papillomavirus (HPV). They may be spread by contact with a wart or shed skin from a wart of another person. New and unusual skin growths should always be evaluated by a dermatologist to rule out skin cancer, especially in persons over fifty or with weakened immune systems.

Over sixty strains of the human papillomavirus have been identified. Common warts (verrucae vulgaris) are typically found on the hands, face, knees, and scalp. Plantar warts are found on the soles of the feet. Perifungal warts are located around the nails.

Digitate warts are found on the scalp. Filiform warts are thin out-growths found around the face and neck. Flat warts occur mainly on the wrists, backs of the hands, and face. The most serious warts are genital warts (condylomata acuminata).

Podophyllin, a plant resin, and chemical medications may be used topically to destroy warts. Warts may also be removed by freezing (cryosurgery), laser surgery, or burning (electrocautery). To prevent the spread of warts, avoid direct contact with them, whether they are on your body or on another person. Refrain-ing from walking barefoot can help prevent plantar warts.

Self-Treatments

- ◆ Garlic remedy: Steep a few cloves in 4 oz castor oil for sev-eral days and apply the mixture topically to warts several times a day. Use gauze or an adhesive strip to cover the wart.
- ◆ Salicylate pad (available in pharmacies): Apply to the wart at bedtime, and remove the following morning. Repeat 5 days in a row. Wart will usually fall off on its own. If not, con-tinue treatment 1 to 2 more weeks. Stop, if no results.
- ◆ Combine equal parts of witch hazel and tinctures of calan-dine, thuja, and blood root, and apply to the wart several times per day. If results are not seen in two weeks, make a paste by combining equal parts of the above tinctures with 50 mcg selenium (break open capsule). Apply paste 2 times daily. This remedy is particularly effective in combination with the salicylate pad remedy (see above).

Professional Treatments

- Astra C (1 to 2 tablets three times a day) and Astra Isatis (2 to 3 tablets three times a day): Use for preventing warts from recurring.
- Clear Heat and Resinall K: Crush 2 tablets Clear Heat and mix with 1 dropperful Resinall K to make a paste. Apply 2 times daily. Cover with an adhesive bandage.
- Moxabustion may help resolve warts, however, regular application is necessary.

Case Study

Julene, a twenty-three-year-old secretary, frequently got warts on her hands. Having them removed was expensive, as this had to be done every few months. All her medical tests were normal. Traditional Chinese medicine diagnosis revealed that her pulse was slightly wiry, and her tongue was red and dry.

We recommended Astra C (1 tablet three times a day) and Astra Isatis (3 tablets three times a day) for one month. She returned commenting that she felt more energetic. Her pulse had become normal, although her tongue was unchanged.

Julene remained on the above protocol for three months. We had her stop the Astra C after three months, and decrease the Astra Isatis (2 tablets three times a day) after two months. She then remained on this formula for over one year. Although not curative, she felt that herbs reduced the number and frequency of occurrences.

Discussion: Astra Isatis has herbs such as astragalus, which enhances the immune system, and isatis, which has antiviral properties. Astra C contains zinc citrate and the Jade Screen Powder formula which helps treat skin conditions. As warts are caused by a virus, the therapeutic strategy was to support the immune system, attack the virus, and nourish the skin.

Wrinkles

Wrinkles form when the skin loses its elasticity—a result of decreased collagen production as we age. Although a certain amount of wrinkling is inevitable with aging, you may reduce the degree of wrinkling with certain skin-protection measures. These include avoiding excessive sun exposure and using a sunscreen with an SPF of at least 15 when you are outside. Other measures such as eating a diet rich in fresh fruits and vegetables, drinking plenty of water, limiting alcohol, refraining from smoking, and avoiding pollutants are also helpful in limiting wrinkle formation.

Repetitive facial expressions can also lead to wrinkling. If you habitually squint, raise your eyebrows, or frown, try to be more aware of these behaviors and reduce their frequency. Facial muscles can also be exercised to tone the skin: Try an exaggerated chewing motion, and stretching the muscles under your chin and on the front of your neck, also with an exaggerated motion. Dermatologists can prescribe Retin-A, which may help smooth wrinkles, but caution is advisable as this treatment can have many side effects.

Self-Treatments

♦ Antioxidant vitamins such as A, C, and E, as well as zinc and selenium have many health benefits and may help preserve the skin (see Chapter Two for therapeutic dosages). Vitamin A (10,000 to 25,000 IU daily) can be helpful for promoting growth of new skin. Vitamin A should be used cautiously during pregnancy; consult your healthcare professional about dosages over 5,000 IU.

- Elastin cream: Helps smooth wrinkles (follow label directions).
- Black currant oil (3,000 mg daily): Helps nourish the skin.
- Silica: Thought to stimulate collagen formation and promote skin elasticity. Silica in the form of colloidal silicic acid used both orally (10 milliliters daily) and topically (follow label directions).
- Horsetail plant: May be taken in capsule form (4,500 mg daily), or drink three cups of tea daily (use 2 teaspoons of horsetail plant per infusion). Such use may promote collagen formation.
- Glucosamine sulfate (1,500 mg per day): Helps regenerate healthy skin and connective tissue.
- Aloe vera gel (follow label directions). Or mix two parts aloe vera gel with one part emu oil with moisturizer, and apply to skin (2 to 3 times daily).
- Pearl Cream: Helps moisturize the skin (follow label directions).

Professional Treatments

Collagenex contains type 2 collagen and grape extract to nourish the skin and nutritionally reduce wrinkles.

Xanthelasma and Xanthoma (Fatty Bumps)

These are yellowish fatty bumps beneath the surface of the skin. Xanthelasmas are one to two millimeters in size and are located on the eyelids near the nose, while xanthomas may be as large as three inches in diameter and commonly appear on the elbows, joints, tendons, knees, hands, feet, or buttocks. Xanthelasmas are associated with elevated cholesterol and triglyceride levels; xanthomas are often an indication of a metabolic disorder such as familial hypercholesterolemia (elevated cholesterol), or conditions such as diabetes, cirrhosis, and some types of cancer.

The primary treatment for xanthelasmas and xanthomas is to treat the underlying disorder. This may involve following a low-cholesterol, low-carbohydrate diet. The growths may also be surgically removed; however, they may reappear if the underlying condition has not been addressed.

Self-Treatments

- Fish oil can be used as part of a healthy cholesterol program (3 g daily).
- Make sure to eat at least 6 to 10 servings of vegetables per day. Plant fiber reduces cholesterol.

Professional Treatments

- Bupleurum Entangled Qi reduces fatty deposits and increases blood circulation. Add Clear Phlegm (1 to 3 tablets three times a day) to reduce phlegm, and phlegm nodules; or Six Gentlemen (3 tablets three times a day) to strengthen the spleen qi.
- Astra Garlic (2 to 3 tablets three times a day): Can also be used to reduce cholesterol.
- Polilipid (1 to 2 tablets two times a day) lowers "bad" LDL cholesterol and raises "good" LDL cholesterol.

Case Study

Carl, a sixty-two-year-old plumber, had xanthomas all over his body. He also had a persistent dry cough, although phlegm was present in the mornings upon waking. Shortness of breath was apparent during and after smoking. His cholesterol level was 210, and his triglycerides were also elevated. He had stopped taking his cholesterol medication because of its side effects. Traditional Chinese medicine diagnosis revealed that Carl's pulse was rapid and choppy, and his tongue was reddish-purple with a thick, gray coating.

Carl was accompanied to our clinic by his daughter, who had been trying to persuade him to quit smoking and drinking, and to stop eating red meat. They came specifically for herbs to reduce the xanthomas. We counseled him that by improving his health and lowering his cholesterol, the bumps would gradually lessen, but that it might not be possible to eliminate them entirely. We recommended Clear Phlegm (1 tablet four times a day), Astra Garlic (2 tablets four times a day), and Quercenol (2 tablets two times a day), an antioxidant formula. We also suggested that he try to reduce his intake of alcohol and sweets (he was accustomed to eating donuts every morning) and to reduce or stop smoking. He was urged to increase his intake of water, fruit, and vegetables. We encouraged him to seek further assistance from his physician if the herbs were not effective in reducing his cholesterol. He was also referred to a dermatologist for consultation about surgical removal of the bumps, and to examine his many moles, age spots, and areas of rough skin.

After three weeks on the herbal formulas, Carl noticed less phlegm, and his daughter thought that he had much more energy and was in a better mood. His pulse was unchanged and his tongue coating was not as thick. After continuing the protocol for another month his cholesterol had dropped to 180 and his triglyceride levels had decreased as well.

After another three months he no longer needed Clear Phlegm. He continued on Quercenol and Astra Garlic at the same dosages. At this point, we recommended Polilipid (2 tablets daily) to further lower his cholesterol. Carl's dermatologist had removed some of the xanthomas, and reported that his skin was aged but had no other abnormalities. Three months later, Carl's cholesterol dropped even more, to 165, and his triglycerides to within high normal range. His pulse had a more regular beat (was less choppy), and his tongue coating was normal.

Chapter Four

Questions and Answers

Why don't you recommend evening primrose oil?

I don't recommend evening primrose oil in the treatment of skin diseases because it is expensive, the studies are inconclusive, and I have not observed it to be effective. Instead I am much more enthusiastic about fish oil, and black currant oil, which can be used as food therapy.

I have red bumps all over my face. I have tried many remedies, but nothing seems to work.

See a dermatologist for a diagnosis. Once you have a firm diagnosis it will be a lot easier to treat.

My dermatologist said there is no evidence that chocolate causes acne.

This may be true in the test tube; however, in contemporary practice there is an absolute link between chocolate and other sugar consumption and acne and other skin conditions. First, chocolate is common allergen, and allergenic substances have been shown to trigger breakouts. Second, chocolate and other sugary foods are considered warming in term of TCM. Therefore, if you want to avoid breakouts, you need to avoid warming foods and beverages. Another problem is that many chocolate products contain dairy products and other additives that can cause, or contribute to skin disorders.

I have psoriasis. I tried some natural therapies and they seemed to help, but it seemed to take too long and I got discouraged. Are natural therapies the best way to go?

Combining a stress reduction and exercise program, a high-potency antioxidant supplement, reducing allergens and sensitivities, eating fresh fish rich in omega-3 fats, and taking appropriate herbs can often bring results in a few months. Gradually over time clients find their skin begins to heal, although major healing may take one year. You may have to make a choice as to how important healthy skin is to you. If it's very important, I'm sure you can make the necessary changes to heal your condition for life.

Aren't bulk herbs more effective than pills?

In order for herbs to be effective, the patient has to take them. At our clinic, we offer clients a choice of administration. The chief advantage of bulk herbs is they can be tailored to the client. The drawback is they take time to be prepared and often do not taste good. Consequently for most of our American clients we recommend pills for long-term administration, and use either pills or teas for short-term administration.

Does the Chinese herb *he shou wu* really work for hair loss?

There are dozens of different kinds of hair loss, and by its reputation *he shou wu* seems to help stop hair loss in some cases, and even restore hair in certain cases. It is by no means one hundred percent effective. I always recommend *he shou wu* to be used in a well-designed herbal formula, as taking *he shou wu* by itself causes loose stools and stomach upset in some patients. Products made in China are not recommended, as they often have additives.

I heard that Chinese herbs are not safe for Americans. Is this true?

It is important to distinguish between bulk herbs, products made in America, and products made overseas. Overseas products often lack quality controls. This has lead to discoveries of products contaminated with drugs and other unsafe ingredients. Bulk Chinese herbs should be administered by trained herbalists as they lead to a strong healing response. Products manufactured in U.S. are made with adequate quality controls and are generally safer than products made overseas or bulk herbs.

My cousin is a hairdresser who works with chemicals all day. Starting last year she developed rashes all over her body. What should she do?

Ideally I would suggest she visit an herbalist or a holistic provider who could suggest liver detoxification strategies. In addition, see if there are less toxic products she could be working with on a daily basis.

What is the best diet for people with inflammatory skin conditions such acne, psoriasis, eczema, rosacea?

It is impossible to prescribe a diet for everyone; however, most people with inflammatory skin conditions do best with a lot of fresh fish such as salmon, plenty of vegetables and fruits—especially berries because they tend to help build up the collagen—and no or extremely low amounts of pro-inflammatory products such as alcohol, sweets, fried foods, and fruit juices (which contain excessive sugars).

What about emu oil?

Emu oil comes from a large ostrich-like bird. It is rich in essential fatty acids. Some people consider it a superior moisturizer, so it can be used externally for any conditions that involves dry skin.

How do you treat tinea versicolor?

This is one of the conditions where I usually recommend Western medicine topically such as nizoral lotion followed by an antifungal herbal formula, coupled with minimizing or eliminating, alcohol, sweets, and refined carbohydrates. Topical drug treatments are quicker, and less messy than herbal options. If you want to go "all natural" I would try the professional formula Biocidin topically. If you cannot get this from your health professional you could try essential oil of tea tree, oregano, or citrus seed oil.

How do you treat hidradenitis?

This condition affects the sweat glands, which are commonly found in the armpits and groin. Deep parts in the skin develop painful swellings that leak pus-like fluids. Odor is a major problem, and people with this disease must bathe or take sponge baths several times per day. The standard treatments are antibiotics, steroids, Accutane (isotretinoin), or skin grafts. Typically symptoms are much worse in hot weather. I have had success with a combination of yin tonics and special stop sweating herbs which can be recommended by a professional herbalist.

How do I know I am getting enough fish oil?

Most clinical studies have shown the benefits using fish oil. Participants have used 3 to 10 grams per day of fish oil. It is important therefore to read the supplements facts box to see how much fish oil you are getting per capsule. For example, a small capsule may only have 500 mg of fish oil, thus you would need to take at least 6 capsules a day to get the minimum dosage. A large capsule may contain up to 1.2 grams (1,200 mg) of fish oil, thus you would have to take 3 capsules a day to get the minimum dosage. One teaspoon of cod liver oil generally contains 5 grams of fish oil, therefore, it is the easiest way to get a therapeutic dosage of fish oil. Cod liver oil in liquid form is easier to digest than fish oil capsules and also contains vitamins A and D. Fish oil may be contraindicated during pregnancy; be sure to consult with your health professional about using fish oil products during pregnancy. Finally it is best to take fish oil products which contain vitamin E or take antioxidants including vitamin E at the same time as taking fish oil. Our recommendation for skin disorders is to eat fresh fish a few times a week, and take 1 to 3 tsp per day of cod liver oil or its equivalent in fish oil capsules.

What do I do about the white patches left from eczema?

White patches are typically not associated with eczema; however, they are associated with other conditions such as vitiligo. We urge you to get a thorough diagnosis from a dermatologist so that your condition can be treated by either standard or complementary approaches.

Are herbs regulated by the FDA?

Yes. The FDA has the right to take unsafe products off the market at any time. The federal and state governments also regulate how products are manufactured.

Should I eat organically?

If you can afford organic foods it's always a good idea. Organic foods reduce the amount of chemicals you consume. Many people find organic foods tastier.

I heard it's not safe to take herbs with drugs?

The best time to take herbs is before a client is on drugs. For example, many Chinese I know try herbs first, if the herbs don't work then they use drugs. I think this is the ideal way to go. Many of us are already taking drugs. It is true that drugs should not be taken at the same time as herbs; it is usually safe to take supplements and drugs at least two hours apart. If you are taking pharmaceuticals, it makes additional sense to see a health professional trained in herbs, for further evaluation.

Is cortisone a steroid?

Cortisone is medically known as corticosteroid. These are topical steroids that are widely sold over the counter for various skin complaints. The chief benefit of steroids is they often initially work quickly and are not messy or smelly. The down side is the tend to loose their effectiveness over time. If taken excessively they can cause the same side effects as oral or injectable steroids, namely increased blood pressure, mood disorders, weight gain, "moon face," and blood sugar problems. If you absolutely must take topical steroids, apply the cream right after a bath, and then wrap the affected area in plastic in order to increase the absorption of the medicine. Many people seek out the help of herbalists and other complementary providers because steroids have stopped working, or they are unhappy with the side effects caused by the medication. Although the majority of people can be helped with approaches mentioned in *Healing Skin Disorders,* it is best to try herbs and natural healing methods first before resorting to drugs.

Digestive Clearing Program*

Digestive Clearing

If your goal is to greatly reduce or eliminate your skin disorders, you must be prepared to examine the foods you are eating. The terms "allergy," "intolerance," and "sensitivity" are used loosely by many people. A *food allergy* actually means that the body's immune system mounts a response to the offending allergen. A true allergy can be diagnosed by laboratory tests, such as with a skin prick, or radioallergosorbent test (RAST). Many persons with digestive disorders have *food sensitivities,* which cannot be detected by a laboratory test, but must be determined through trial and error. In addition to skin disorders, food sensitivities can cause abdominal cramping, diarrhea, constipation, intestinal gas, bloating, vomiting, nausea, ulcers, fatigue, joint pain, muscle aches, edema, headaches, migraines, depression, anxiety, respiratory

---

*Use this program to determine if the foods you are eating may be causing skin reactions. Adapted from *Healing Digestive Disorders* by Andrew Gaeddert.

difficulties, hyperactivity, and attention disorders.

Why are we so sensitive? We are exposed to thousands of chemicals our ancestors were never exposed to: pollutants, residues from fertilizer and pesticides, additives, preservatives, flavoring agents, among others. The earliest nutritionist was our nose and tongue. The foods we needed smelled good. When we had enough to eat, the food no longer appealed to our taste. With the advent of food processing, our senses of taste and smell were no longer reliable. And when the refrigerator and modern transportation came into being, foods that are genetically intolerable are now available.

Our ancestors ate what was available in their environments. The Native American Indian of the plains who was severely allergic to buffalo, the Asian who couldn't eat rice, or the Irish who couldn't eat potatoes, simply died. People then were much more active, so sensitivities were not taken into consideration. Everyday was a struggle for survival. When chased by wild animals, or fighting a warring tribe, one does not concern oneself about abdominal pain or constipation!

It is no wonder that millions of us have digestive disorders. We are bombarded with stress and don't exercise; we are exposed to foods and chemicals our digestive systems weren't designed to handle; and many of us were not breast-fed. Breastfeeding seems to protect us from developing allergies and sensitivities.

Another problem that persons with digestive difficulties face are food cravings. Often, the cravings are for foods that one is actually sensitive to. I have counseled many digestive and respiratory patients who make statements like: "I must have cereal and milk every morning." Parts of the treatment involve refraining from the food one craves, in this case cereal and milk, for at least two weeks. Other unhealthy cravings may be dairy, alcohol, fruit, sweets, fructose, tomatoes, soy, and greasy foods. When the food cravings are based on emotional difficulties, psychological counseling may also be helpful.

Digestive Meal Plan

The purpose of the digestive clearing meal plan is to help you identify foods that are problematic for your body. If you follow this plan faithfully you can greatly reduce or eliminate your digestive symptoms. You should plan about one month for your digestive clearing program. I recommend that you do not begin when holidays, vacations, or celebrations are planned. It is very much like quitting smoking: you need to make a plan.

It is possible that you may feel worse for the first few days of clearing, but don't cheat! It will be worth it in the long run. As I do not believe in making drastic changes, the first two weeks are a "winding down" period, the next two weeks consist of taking in foods that are not commonly known to cause sensitivities, followed by a reintroduction phase. It is essential that you keep a journal during this process. Once you have located a food you are sensitive to, it may be possible through the use of herbs and other dietary supplements to build up your system so that you can occasionally incorporate it back into your diet. You may notice that you feel so much better without consuming a formerly craved food, that it is not worthwhile to reincorporate it. Chapter Two has a list of foods that have been known to produce reactions in digestive patients.

For the first two weeks, you should begin reducing and then eliminating "not allowed" foods from your diet. If you are eating any of these foods more than once a day, you should cut down your consumption by 50 percent the first day, then eliminate it by the end of the second week. All food you eat should be cooked. This will reduce food reactivity. Locate a health food store or supermarket where you can obtain fresh foods and foods without additives, pesticides, antibiotics, and hormones. Drink at least 64 ounces of filtered or spring water, or herbal teas. You may place a slice of cucumber, lemon, or lime wedge in the water to make it tastier. You should maintain the increased water or herbal tea intake throughout the clearing and reintroduction phase. Whenever possible, drink hot water; *never drink ice water.* If taken from the refrigerator, let water reach room temperature.

I have provided a sample meal plan below. Feel free to improvise as long as you are eating the allowable foods. The not-allowed list is not exhaustive, so if the food is not on the allowed list, don't eat it! Also included are recommendations for the use of supplements which should be started during the preparation phase, or after clearing is completed.

Protein

Allowed

Beef, pork, lamb, venison, chicken, turkey, duck, goose, rabbit, pheasant, quail, or other game. Fresh fish.

Not Allowed

Shellfish, prepared fish (such as breaded or fish sticks), prepared or preserved meats such as bacon, sausages, hot dogs, cold cuts.

Preparation

Boiled, baked, broiled, poached. Avoid deep frying.

Vegetables

Allowed

Most. Limit potatoes to 1 per day.

Not Allowed

Soybean, tomatoes, cabbage, broccoli, cauliflower, mushrooms, brussels sprouts, beans, peas, lentils. These should be the first foods to be reintroduced.

Preparation

Try to use only fresh vegetables. Frozen vegetables may be used when in a pinch. All vegetables should be steamed or boiled. Light stir-frying with olive oil is suitable. Spray olive oil or use a maximum of 1 tablespoon per serving of extra virgin olive oil. After two weeks begin to use salad dressings with olive, canola, hemp, or flax oils (no more than 1 tablespoon of oil per serving). Add vinegar a few days later.

Fruits

Allowed

None during the digestive clearing phase. Thereafter, begin with bananas, pears, apples, kiwi fruit, mangoes, papaya, pomegranates, passion fruit, guava, and melons. Blueberries, strawberries, raspberries and other fruit may be added later, after you have tested the previous fruits.

Starch and Grains

Allowed

Rice, millet, amaranth, tapioca, buckwheat, and quinoa. During the reintroduction phase, add gluten-containing foods (oats, barley, rye, spelt), yeast-free muffins and crackers before adding breads.

Nuts

Eliminate during the clearing phase. During the reintroduction phase, you can start incorporating nuts and nut butters, however, peanuts and peanut butter should be tested last.

Seasoning

Sea salt, pepper, herbs and spices, if they are used alone (i.e., don't use combination seasonings).

Beverages

Filtered water, spring water, herbal tea. Only black or green tea may be used during the preparation phase to reduce or eliminate caffeine cravings. During the reintroduction phase, you can experiment with carbonated water if desired. Fruit juices should be reintroduced last and should only be used half strength or more diluted.

Prohibited Foods

Any food not on the above list, including but not limited to dairy products (milk, cream, butter, cheese, yogurt, ice cream), eggs, sweets, yeast, pastry, prepared or instant food, vinegar, marmite (yeast extract), alcoholic beverages, canned foods, horseradish, bouillon, bread, bagels, pizza, rolls, chips, salad dressing, desserts, fruits and fruit juices, ice drinks, soda, and uncooked foods.

If You Still Have Symptoms

The digestive clearing plan gives your body a vacation. Not all vacations are great one hundred percent of the time. However, when we look back, we can say it was worth it. Therefore, it is realistic to expect withdrawal symptoms for the first few days. For example, on a vacation you may miss your friends or colleagues from work. Similarly, on the clearing plan, you may miss your morning cup of coffee or your gooey sweet roll. If after a week you do not feel fewer symptoms and more energy and mental clarity, it is possible that you could have sensitivities to the digestive clearing diet. If you have eliminated all the items listed as not allowed, try meats that you have not eaten before. The same applies to vegetables. Also, have you been cheating? Check your food diary. Is there something that you ate on the run? One of my clients, Jessica, was not experiencing any improvement on the clearing program; it turns out she had not given up alcohol.

It is also possible that chemicals such as perfume, airplane glue, sprays, lighter fluid, or even particleboard may be causing your symptoms. In this case, you should consult a health professional specializing in environmental allergies. In addition, changes in barometric pressure, particularly as the weather becomes more humid, have been known to trigger joint pain and other symptoms.

An elimination diet of lamb, pears, yams, sweet potatoes, millet, rice, and hypoallergenic protein powder (available from holistic health professionals) can be used as an alternative to the Digestive Clearing Plan, however, professional supervision is recommended. Another diet known as the Rare Foods Diet can be selected. This involves eating only foods you have never eaten before, such as ostrich, quinoa, amaranth, and other exotic foods.

Meal Plan With Supplementation

One half-hour before meals take an acidophilus/bifidus product in capsule or powder form. Take a separate product with FOS. Follow instructions on the bottle carefully. The natural therapy section (Chapter Three) has recommended brands.

One half-hour before breakfast

- Acidophilus/bifidus

Breakfast

- Rice or millet porridge
- Antioxidant vitamin, folic acid, and B12

Snack

- Sweet potato, yam, acorn squash, artichoke, rice cakes

Lunch

- Homemade beef, chicken, or turkey vegetable soup
- Meat or fish
- Steamed vegetables and rice
- Antioxidant vitamin, folic acid, and B12

Snack

- Sweet potato, yam, acorn squash, artichoke, rice cakes

Dinner

- Meat, fish, or homemade soup
- Vegetable—steamed, boiled, or stir-fried (1 tablespoon extra virgin olive oil per serving)
- Allowable grains
- Sweet potato, yam, acorn squash
- Pasta made from quinoa or Jerusalem artichoke

Beverages

- Filtered water
- Herbal tea: Pau d' Arco, peppermint, ginger (with cold signs), most other herbal teas

Bedtime

- Acidophilus/bifidus
- Healing bath (see Chapter Two)

Reintroduction Phase

After two weeks begin reintroducing foods in the indicated order. A new food can be introduced every four hours. If symptoms occur, put that food on your list of items to be tested at a later date. If you were under stress, fatigued, or having your period when testing, put on your "possible sensitivity" list and retest in one month or so. Start with the vegetables indicated. See if raw or cooked makes a difference, starting with one serving of raw vegetables per day. If this agrees with you, try making homemade oil and herb dressing. If this agrees with you, add vinegar in a few days.

Next, introduce whole fruit, then oatmeal, yeast-free muffins, followed by crackers, and all other foods. Put off processed foods and multi-ingredient foods as long as possible as they make identifying sensitivities more difficult. If you follow this plan under the guide of a health professional, he/she may suggest protein powders and added nutrients. There are pros and cons of adding vitamins to this program. In general, if you can, high quality, hypoallergenic vitamins are recommended. They will help you heal your GI system faster (see Chapter Three). The disadvantage of using vitamins at this point is that they may mask symptoms; but I believe that the advantages of vitamins far outweigh this one disadvantage.

If constipation occurs while undergoing this program, supplement with flax seed, or products containing rice bran, ground flax seeds, flax oil, guar gum, and other soluble fibers. You can also increase your consumption of vegetables and add prunes. If your stools are looser while following this program, temporarily reduce the vegetables (and fruits, if you are into the reintroduction phase) and introduce them more slowly. If you are still having problems, seek the help of a health professional.

I have personally found this plan to be very beneficial. My clients and other health professionals agree that giving their digestive systems a break is very helpful. Admittedly, it is more difficult for vegetarians. It may be possible to obtain protein in the form of protein shakes. However, many of these products have common allergens and have ingredients such as algae and spirulina that are hard to digest. Hypoallergenic protein powders can be obtained through holistic professionals.

Digestive Clearing Worksheet

This worksheet is to help you identify your food sensitivities.

- What foods can't I live without?

_____

_____

_____

_____

_____

- What foods lead to symptoms, or do I suspect I may be sensitive to? (Do not edit.)

_____

_____

_____

_____

- What major dietary change have I undertaken? Did that make my digestion better or worse?

_____

_____

_____

_____

_____

• What foods or beverages do I have more than once per day?

_____

_____

_____

_____

_____

• What do I like to do that does not involve eating?

_____

_____

_____

_____

_____

_____

_____

_____

_____

_____

_____

Additional Formulas

Bupleurum Entangled Qi Formula

Therapeutic Actions
1. Treats breast lumps.
2. Useful in treatments for uterine fibroids and ovarian, vulvar, or cervical cysts.
3. May also be used as an adjunct to post-breast cancer treatment.
4. Can also treat depression.

Chinese Therapeutic Effects
- Vitalizes Qi and Blood Circulation
- Clears Heat and Toxins
- Resolves Phlegm

Ingredients: Bupleurum Root, *Chai Hu;* Tang-kuei Root, *Dang Gui;* Blue Citrus Fruit, *Qing Pi;* Prunella Herb, *Xia Ku Cao;* Salvia Root, *Dan Shen;* Tricosanthes Root, *Tian Hua Fen;* Vaccaria Fruit, *Wang Bu Liu Xing;* White Peony Root, *Bai Shao;* Cyperus Rhizome, *Xiang Fu;* Ligusticum Root, *Chuan Xiong;* Fritillaria Bulb, *Chuan Bei Mu;* Dandelion Herb, *Pu Gong Ying;* Red Peony Root, *Chi Shao*

Channel Flow

Therapeutic Actions

1. Has pain relieving and relaxant properties.
2. Helps relieve joint, muscle, abdominal and gynecological pain and cramping.
3. Treats headache, arthritis, and fibromyalgia, especially when used with other formulas.

Chinese Therapeutic Effects

- Regulates Qi and Blood
- Warms the Channels

Ingredients: Corydalis Rhizome, *Yan Hu Suo;* Angelica Root, *Bai Zhi;* Peony Root, *Bai Shao;* Cinnamon Twig, *Gui Zhi;* Tang-kuei Root, *Dang Gui;* Salvia Root, *Dan Shen;* Myrrh Resin, *Mo Yao;* Frankincense Gum, *Ru Xiang;* Licorice Root, *Gan Cao*

Clearing

Therapeutic Actions

1. Addresses chronic vaginal and urethral irritation and inflammation.
2. May be used for chronic bladder infections.
3. Treats chronic diarrhea with Yin deficiency.
4. Treats stomatitis (mouth sores).

Chinese Therapeutic Effects

- Clears Heat from the Heart, Lungs, Liver, Stomach, and Bladder

- Tonifies Spleen Qi and Resolves Dampness
- Circulates and Nourishes the Blood

Ingredients: Lotus Seed, *Lian Zi;* Ophiopogon Tuber, *Mai Men Dong;* Poria Sclerotium, *Fu Ling;* White Ginseng Root, *Jilin Ren Shen;* Plantaginis Seed, *Che Qian Zi;* Scutellaria Root, *Huang Qin;* Smilax Rhizome, *Tu Fu Ling;* Astragalus Root, *Huang Qi;* Lycium Bark, *Di Gu Pi;* Moutan Rootbark, *Mu Dan Pi;* Red Peony Root, *Chi Shao;* Licorice Root, *Gan Cao*

Clear Heat

Therapeutic Actions

1. Take for viral, bacterial, and fungal infections. Especially designed for persons with HIV infections. May be used also for Chronic Immune Dysfunction Syndrome (CIDS), Chronic Fatigue Syndrome (CFS), chronic herpes, viral warts, and other chronic viral infections.
2. Useful for pain with heat signs.

Chinese Therapeutic Effects

- Clears Heat and Cleans Toxin
- Tonifies Kidney Essence
- Dissolves Phlegm Nodules
- Tonifies Lung Yin

Ingredients: Isatis Extract Leaf and Root, *Ban Lan Gen* and *Da Qing Ye;* Old-enlandia Herb, *Bai Hua She She Cao;* Lonicera Flower, *Jin Yin Hua;* Prunella Herb, *Xia Ku Cao;* Andrographis Rhizome, *Chuan Xin Lian;* Laminaria Leaf, *Kun Bu;* Viola Herb and Root, *Zi Hua Di Ding;* Cordyceps Fruiting Body, *Dong Chong Xia Cao;* Licorice Root, *Gan Cao*

Coptis Purge Fire Formula

Therapeutic Actions

1. Treats intense, acute, localized inflammations, skin eruptions such as hives, sore throat, strep throat, eye and ear infections, nasal and sinus infections, herpes simplex

outbreaks, pelvic inflammatory disease, tooth abscess, oral ulcers, and nasal infections, mouth ulcers.

2. Treats chronic liver fire conditions, chronic skin eruptions (eczema), facial flushing, red eyes, migraine headaches, urinary tract infections.
3. Treats constipation associated with illnesses and high fevers.
4. Useful for hot flashes.

Chinese Therapeutic Effects

♦ Purges Fire and Toxins
♦ Dries Dampness

Ingredients: Coptis Root, *Huang Lian;* Lophatherum Herb, *Dan Zhu Ye;* Bupleurum Root, *Chai Hu;* Rehmannia Root, *Sheng Di Huang;* Tang Kuei Root, *Dang Gui;* Peony Root, *Bai Shao;* Akebia Trifoliata Root, *Mu Tong;* Anemarrhena Rhizome, *Zhi Mu;* Phellodendron Bark, *Huang Bai;* Gentiana Root, *Long Dan Cao;* Alisma Rhizome, *Ze Xie;* Plantago Seed, *Che Qian Zi;* Scute Root, *Huang Qin;* Sophora Root, *Ku Shen;* Forsythia Fruit, *Lian Qiao;* Gardenia Fruit, *Zhi Zi;* Licorice Root, *Gan Cao*

Coriolus PS

Therapeutic Actions

1. Japanese research shows that this medicinal mushroom extract has anti-tumor effects and stimulates natural killer (NK) cells. Used in conjunction with chemo and radiation therapy, Coriolus has been found to be instrumental in helping increase cancer survival rates.
2. Stimulates production of killer T cells and tumor necrosis factor (TNF); activates macrophage function.
3. Also used as adjunct for hepatitis, lung infections.

Ingredients: Coriolus Versicolor, *Yun Zhi;* extract containing 25% polysaccharides

Drain Dampness

Therapeutic Actions

1. Diuretic, diaphoretic.
2. Primary indications are edema, difficulty in urination, sensation of heaviness.
3. Secondary considerations are thirst, headaches, vomiting, foamy saliva, pulsations below the naval.
4. In China this formula may be used to treat chronic nephritic edema, acute gastritis, cardiac edema, ascites due to liver cirrhosis, urinary retention, scrotal hydrocele, acute enteritis with diarrhea, cholera, prostaic hypertrophy.
5. According to *Formulas and Strategies* this formula may be effective for nephritis, renal failure, ascites from liver cirrhosis, Menieres disease, hepatitis, gastroptosis, gastrectasis, gastroenteritis, enteritis, genitourinary infections, neurogenic bladder syndrome, and hydrocele.

Chinese Therapeutic Effects

◆ Stagnation of Water and Dampness in the body
◆ Strengthen the Spleen

Ingredients: Alisma Rhizome, *Ze Xie;* Poria Sclerotium, *Fu Ling;* Polyporus Sclerotium, *Zhu Ling;* Cinnamon Twig, *Gui Zhi;* White Atractylodes Root, *Bai Zhu*

Flavonex

Therapeutic Actions

1. Used for prevention of degenerative cardiovascular diseases.
2. Used to promote cerebral functions.
3. Treats circulatory-related problems, neuropathy, arthritis, menstrual disorders, poor mental functions, gastric ulcer, colitis, sciatica.
4. May be used for cardiovascular disease.

Chinese Therapeutic Effects

- ◆ Dilates Peripheral and Coronary Blood Vessels
- ◆ Promotes Blood Circulation
- ◆ Nourish and Astringe Essence

Ingredients: Pueraria Root, *Ge Gen;* Ilex Root, *Mao Dong Qing;* Salvia Root, *Dan Shen;* Lonicera Flower, *Jin Yin Hua;* Eucommia Bark, *Du Zhong;* Acorus Rhizome, *Shi Chang Pu;* Cistanche Herb, *Rou Cong Rong;* Ho-shou-wu Root, *He Shou Wu;* Morus Fruit, *Sang Shen;* Rosa Fruit, *Jin Ying Zi;* Lycium Fruit, *Gou Qi Zi;* Zizyphus Seed, *Suan Zao Ren;* Tang-kuei Root, *Dang Gui;* Schizandra Fruit, *Wu Wei Zi;* Gingko biloba Leaf Extract, *Yin Guo Ye;* 24% Flavonoids; 6% Lactones

Mobility 2

Therapeutic Actions

1. Treats severe chronic arthritis or rheumatism characterized by inflammatory processes and stagnation of blood flow in the joints.
2. Treats gout, sciatica, lumbago.
3. Treats edema.

Chinese Therapeutic Effects

- ◆ Relieves the Surface
- ◆ Promotes the Flow of Water
- ◆ Dispels Wind-Damp
- ◆ Vitalizes Blood Circulation

Ingredients: Red Peony Root, *Chi Shao;* Tang kuei Root, *Dang Gui;* Ligusticum Radix, *Chuan Xiong;* Rehmannia Root, *Shu Di Huang;* Persica Kernel, *Tao Ren;* Atractylodes Rhizome, *Bai Zhu;* Poria Sclerotium, *Fu Ling;* Citrus Rind, *Chen Pi;* Siler Root, *Fang Feng;* Vitex Seed, *Man Jing Zi;* Gentiana Root, *Qin Jiao;* Achyranthes Root, *Niu Xi;* Chianghuo Rhizome, *Qiang Huo;* Clematis Root, *Wei Ling Xian;* Ginger Rhizome, *Gan Jiang;* Angelica Root, *Bai Zhi;* Licorice Root, *Gan Cao*

Nine Flavor Tea

Therapeutic Actions

1. Treats chronic and recurrent sore throat with lymphatic swelling.
2. Treats oral sores accompanied by thirst and insomnia.
3. Treats a symptom combination that includes facial flushing, afternoon fevers, chronic inflammation, burning soles and palms, nightsweats, blurred vision, dizziness, tinnitus, and impotence.

Chinese Therapeutic Effects

- Nourishes Liver, Kidney, Stomach, Spleen Yin
- Clears Stomach Heat and Heart Fire
- Tonifies Kidney and Spleen Qi

Ingredients: Rehmannia Root, *Shu Di Huang & Sheng Di Huang;* Dioscorea Rhizome, *Shan Yao;* Poria Sclerotium, *Fu Ling;* Cornus Fruit, *Shan Zhu Yu;* Moutan Root Bark, *Mu Dan Pi;* Alisma Rhizome, *Ze Xie;* Scrophularia Root, *Xuan Shen;* Ophiopogon Tuber, *Mai Men Dong*

Quercenol

Typical Applications: Antioxidant

Ingredients (2 tablets): Quercetin (400 mg), Silybum marianum (250 mg), Proanthocyanidins (125 mg), Green tea polyphenols (150 mg), Mixed carotenoids (30 mg), Vitamin E (300 IU), Vitamin C (500 mg), Zinc (10 mg), Selenium (100 mcg).

Quiet Digestion

Therapeutic Actions

1. Treats gastric distress, including abdominal pain, sudden and violent cramping, nausea, vomiting, diarrhea, regurgitation, gastric hyperactivity, abdominal distension, poor appetite, and intestinal gas.

2. Treats gastroenteritis, bacterial or viral.
3. Treats motion sickness, hangover, and the effects of jet lag.
4. Difficulty absorbing food.

Chinese Therapeutic Effects

♦ Disperses Wind and Dampness
♦ Resolves Spleen Dampness and Regulates the Stomach
♦ Resolves Phlegm

Ingredients: Poria Sclerotium, *Fu Ling;* Coix Seed, *Yi Yi Ren;* Shen Chu Herb, *Shen Qu;* Magnolia Bark, *Hou Po;* Angelica Root, *Bai Zhi;* Pueraria Root, *Ge Gen;* Red Atractylodes Rhizome, *Cang Zhu;* Jurinea Root, *Mu Xiang;* Pogostemon Herb, *Huo Xiang;* Oryza Sprout, *Gu Ya;* Trichosanthes Root, *Tian Hua Fen;* Chrysanthemum Flower, *Ju Hua;* Halloysite, *Chi Shi Zhi;* Citrus Rind, *Ju Hong;* Mentha Herb, *Bo He*

Vagistatin

Therapeutic Actions

1. Normalizes dysbiosis of vagina due to fungus, yeast, bacteria, virus, and protozoa.
2. Normalizes epithelial tissue in early stages of cervical dysplasia.
3. Attacks human papilloma virus (HPV).
4. Treats vaginal discharge.
5. May also be used for colitis, diaper rash, and oral thrush.

Chinese Therapeutic Effects

♦ Dispels Toxic Heat and Damp-Heat of Vagina
♦ Invigorates Blood to Regenerate Tissue

Ingredients: Isatis Extract Leaf & Root, *Ban Lan Gen & Da Qing Ye;* Phellodendron Bark, *Huang Bai;* Salvia Root, *Dan Shen;* Artemesia Herb, *Qing Hao;* Houttuynia Herb, *Yu Xing Cao;* Cnidium Fruit, *She Chuang Zi;* Whole Agrimony, *Xian He Cao*

Skin Acupoints

Acne

GB 38 *(Yangfu)*, GB 41 *(Zulinqi)*, GB 43 *(Xiaxi)*, Li 2 *(Xingjian)*.

Boils (furuncles)

B 54 *(Weizhong)*—needle or bloodlet, Gv 10 *(Lingtai)*, Gv 12 *(Shenzhu)*, LI 4 *(Hegu)*.

Canker Sores

Co 23 *(Lianquan)*, Gv 27 *(Duiduan)*, LI 4 *(Hegu)*, P 8 *(Laogong)*, SI 1 *(Shaoze)*, TB 5 *(Waiguan)*, M-HN-20 *(Jinjin Yuye)*.

Eczema

GB 30 *(Huantiao)*, Gv 14 *(Dazhui)*, H 7 *(Shenmen)*, LI 11 *(Dazhui)*, Sp 6 *(Sanyinjiao)*, Sp10 *(Xuehai)*, St 36 *(Zusanli)*.

Ear points: Lung, Neurogate, Shenmen.

Infants and children: acupressure may be used for infants and young children: Co 12 *(Zhongwan)*, St 25 *(Tianshu)*, St 12 *(Quepen)*, St 14 *(Kufang)*.

Wind–damp type: LI 11 *(Qichi)*, Sp 10 *(Xuehai)*, Gv 14 *(Dazhui)*, Gv 13 *(Taodao)*. For predominant dampness, add Sp 9 *(Yinlingquan)*, Co 9 *(Shuifen)*.

Ear points: Corresponding body areas; Lung, Adrenal, Adrenal Gland, Shenmen.

Frostbite

Warm affected areas with moxa for 15 minutes 2 to 3 times daily.

Hives (Urticaria)

Gv 14 *(Dazhui)*, LI 11 *(Quchi)*, Sp 6 *(Sanyinjiao)*, Sp 9 *(Yinlingquan)*, Sp10 *(Xuehai)*, S 36 *(Zusanli)*.

Ear points: Lung, Adrenal, Shenmen, Endocrine.

Itching

B 16 *(Dushu)*, GB 31 *(Fengshi)*, GB 34 *(Yanlingquan)*, Li 5 *(Ligou)*, St 15 *(Wuyi)*.

For redness: Add TB 3 *(Zhongzhu)*.

For dampness: Add B 28 *(Pangguangshu)*.

Lymphedema

Co 5 *(Shimen)*, Co 6 *(Qihai)*, Co 7 *(Yinjiao)*, Co 9 *(Shuifen)*, Gv 20 *(Baihui)*, P 2 *(Tianquan)*, P 3 *(Quze)*, Sp 6 *(Sanyinjiao)*, Sp 9 *(Yinlingquan)*, St 36 *(Zusanli)*.

Shingles (Herpes zoster)

TB 5 *(Waiguan)*, LI 11 *(Quchi)*, Sp10 *(Xuehai)*, Sp 6 *(Sanyinjiao)*, Li 3 *(Taichong)*. Consult dermatome chart.

Sunburn

Co12 *(Zhongwan)*, Gv 14 *(Dazhui)*, LI 4 *(Hegu)*, LI 11 *(Quchi)*, Li 3 *(Taichong)*, P 6 *(Neiguan)*, S 44 *(Neiting)*, Sp 4 *(Gongsun)*.

Sweating

Excessive sweating: LI 4 *(Hegu)*, Li 1 *(Dadun)*, L 1 *(Zhongfu)*, L 7 *(Lieque)*, Sp15 *(Daheng)*.

Lack of sweating: B 13 *(Feishu)*, B 14 *(Jueyinshu)*, B 29 *(Zhongl, shu)*, B 67 *(Zhiyin)*, GB 11 *(Touqiaoyin)*, GB 44 *(Zuqiaoyin)*, Gv 13 *(Taodao)*, Gv 15 *(Yamen)*, LI 4 *(Hegu)*, S 12 *(Quepen)*, S 39 *(Xiajushu)*.

Night sweats: H 6 *(Yinxi)*, SI 3 *(Houxi)*, B 13 *(Feishu)*, B 15 *(Xinshu)*, B 17 *(Geshu)*, Gv 14 *(Dazhui)*, K 2 *(Rangu)*, K 7 *(Fuliu)*, K 8 *(Jiaoxin)*, M-HN-30 *(Bailao)*, TB 5 *(Waiguan)*.

Warts

Apply moxa to wart for 5 minutes, 2 to 3 times daily. Also needle St 36 *(Zusanli)*, LI 4 *(Hegu)*, Sp 10 *(Xuehai)*.

Appendix D

Resource Guide

For further information, a list of practitioners in your area who recommend herbs, and/or information about seminars or our upcoming newsletter, write to the author:

Andrew Gaeddert
c/o Get Well Clinic
8001A Capwell Drive
Oakland, CA 94621
510-635-9778   Fax: 510-639-9140
E-mail: GWFClinic@aol.com

The following are organizations or agencies that offer information and support to persons with skin conditions.

American Lupus Society
3914 Del Amo Boulevard, Suite 922
Torrance, CA 90503
310-542-8891   or   1-800-331-1802
Charlean Wakefield

American Skin Association

150 East 58th Street, 33rd floor
New York, NY 10155-0002
212-753-8260
1-800-499-SKIN
Fax 212-688-6547
Joyce Weidler, Managing Director

Foundation for Ichthyosis and Related Skin Types (F.I.R.S.T.)

P.O. Box 669
Ardmore, PA 19003-0669
1-800-545-3286
e-mail: 74722.1571@compuserve.com

Gluten Intolerance Group of North America (Dermatitis Herpetiformis)

P.O. Box 23503
Seattle, WA 98102-0353
206-325-6980

Lupus Foundation of America, Inc.

1300 Picard Drive, Suite 200
Rockville, MD 20850-4503
301-670-9292
1-800-558-0121
Fax 301-670-9486
John Huber, Executive Director
Barbara Butler, Board of Directors
www.lupus.org/lupus

National Alopecia Areata Foundation
710 "C" St., Suite 11
San Rafael, CA 94901
Ph: 415-456-4644
www.alopeciaareata.com

National Arthritis and Musculoskeletal and Skin Disease Information Clearinghouse
National Institutes of Health
1 AMS Circle
Bethesda, MD 20892-3675

National Cancer Institute
Office of Communications
National Institute for Health
9000 Rockville Pike
Building 31, Room 10A31
Bethesda, MD 20892
301-496-6631
1-800-4-CANCER Cancer Information Service
Fax 301-402-4945
Paul Van Nevel, Associate Director

National Eczema Association for Science and Education
1220 SW Morrison, Suite 433
Portland, OR 97205
503-228-4430
800-818-7546
www.eczema-assn.org

National Foundation for Vitiligo and Pigment Disorders

9032 South Normandy Drive
Centerville, OH 45459
513-885-5739

National Herpes Hotline

919-361-8485

National Psoriasis Foundation

6600 SW 92nd Ave., Suite 300
Portland, OR 97223
503-244-7404 or 1-800-723-9166
www.psoriasis.org

National Registry for Ichthyosis and Related Disorders

Dermatology, Box 356524
University of Washington
Seattle, WA 98195-6524
Geoff Hamill, R.N., Registry Coordinator
e-mail: geoff@u.washington.edu
Philip Fleckman, M.D., Principal Investigator
e-mail: fleck@u.washington.edu
1-800-595-1265

National Rosacea Society

220 South Cook Street, Suite 201
Barrington, IL 60010
708-382-8971
Fax 708-382-5567
Suzanne Corr, Director

National Sjögren Syndrome Association

21630 North 19th Avenue
Phoenix, AZ 85027
602-516-0787
Fax 602-516-0111

National Vitiligo Foundation

P.O. Box 6337
611 South Fleishel Ave.
Tyler, TX 75701
Ph: 903-531-0074

Obsessive-Compulsive Foundation

337 Notch Hill Rd.
North Branford, CT 06471
203-315-2190
www.ocfoundation.org

Sarcoidosis Family Aid and Medical Research Foundation

460 Central Avenue
East Orange, NJ 07018
201-399-3644
1-800-203-6429
Geneva Ausley, President and Founder

Scleroderma Info Exchange, Inc.

150 Hines Farm Road
Cranston, RI 02921
401-943-3909
Nancy D. Hersy, Executive Director

Xeroderma Pigmentosum Society
57 Sleight Plass Road
Poughkeepsie, NY 12603
914-473-4735
e-mail: jcqc92a@prodigy.com
Caren J. Mahar, Director

The following organization helps protect the freedom of Americans to use vitamins and herbal products.

Citizens for Health
2031 16th Street
Boulder, CO 80302
303-417-0772

Notes

1. Broda O. Barnes and Lawrence Galton, *Hypothyroidism: The Unsuspected Illness,* Harper & Row, New York, NY, 1976.
2. *Let's Live,* April 1999, p. 43.
3. Murray, Michael T. *The Healing Power of Herbs,* Prima Publishing, 1992, 1995, p. 177.
4. *Let's Live,* March 2000, p. 44.
5. Baumgartner, M. "Allergic medicine, 1998" *Health Notes,* Fall 1999, pp. 158–61.
6. Worwood, Valerie Ann. *The Complete Book of Essential Oils & Aromatherapy,* New World Library, 1991.
7. Perricone, Nicholas, M.D. *The Wrinkle Cure.* Warner Books, New York, NY.
8. Murray, Michael T. *Encyclopedia of Nutritional Supplements,* Prima Publishing, 1996, p. 265.
9. Ibid. Murray, p. 187.
10. Santucci, B., Critaudo, A., Mehraban, M., et al. "ZNSO4 treatment of NiSO4 positive patients." *Contact Dermatitis,* 1999; 40: 281–2.
11. Altmeyer, P. J., Matthes, U., Pawlak, F., Hoffman, K., Frosch, P. J., Ruppert, P., Wassilew, S.W., et al. "Anti-psoriatic effect of fumaric acid derivatives. Results of

multicenter double blind study in 100 patients." *J AM Academy of Dermatology,* 1994; 30 (6): 977–81.

12. Kieffer, M. E., Efsen, J. "Imedeen in the treatment of photoaged skin: an efficacy and safety trial over 12 months." *J Euro Acad. Dermatol Venereol* 1998 ep: 11(2): 129–36.

13. Lassus, A., Jeskanen, L., Happonen, H. P., Santalahti, J. "Imedeen for the treatment of degenerated skin in females," *J Int Med Res* 1991 Mar–Apr; 19(2): 147–152.

14. Griffith, R. S., DeLong, D. C., Nelson, J. D. "Relation of arginine/lysine antagonism to herpes simplex growth in tissue culture." *Chemotherapy* 27(3): 209–213, 1981.

15. Worm, W. "Clinical relevance of food additives in adult patients with atopic dermatitis." *Clinical Experiments in Allergy,* 30: 407–414, 2000.

16. *Natural Health,* April 1999, p. 46.

17. Balch, James, and Balch, Phyllis. *Prescription for Nutritional Healing.*

18. White, L. "Remedies for vitiligo." *Nutrition Science News,* 4(7): 350, 1999.

19. Run, R. "Treatment of 117 cases of vitiligo with wumei tincture." *Shiyong Zhongyiyao Zazhi,* 16(8): 32, 2000.

Bibliography

Bensky, Dan, and Andrew Gamble. *Chinese Herbal Medicine: Materia Medica Revised Edition*. Seattle, WA: Eastland Press, Inc., 1993.

Blumenthal, Mark, Alicia Goldberg, and Josef Brinckmann. *Herbal Medicine*. Newton, MA: Integrative Medicine Communications, 2000.

Castleman, Michael. *The Healing Herbs*. New York, NY: Bantam Books, 1991.

Crook, William. *The Yeast Connection*. New York, NY: Random House, Inc., 1986.

Dharmananda, Subhuti. *A Bag of Pearls*. Portland, OR: I.T.M. and Preventive Health Care, 2000.

Fitzpatrick, James, and John Aeling. *Dermatology Secrets in Color, Second Edition*. Philadelphia, PA: Hanley & Belfus, Inc., 2001.

Gaeddert, Andrew. *Chinese Herbs in the Western Clinic*. Berkeley, CA: North Atlantic Books, 1994.

Gaeddert, Andrew. *Clinical Handbook, Second Edition.* Oakland, CA: Professional Health Concerns, 2002.

Gaeddert, Andrew. *Digestive Health NOW.* Berkeley, CA: North Atlantic Books, 2002.

Gaeddert, Andrew. *Healing Digestive Disorders.* Berkeley, CA: North Atlantic Books, 1998.

Kaptchuk, Ted. *K'an Herbals Formula Guide.* Scott's Valley, CA: K'an Herbals, 1998.

Kirschmann, Gayla, and John Kirschmann. *Nutrition Almanac, Fourth Edition.* New York, NY: McGraw-Hill, 1996.

Krohn, Jacqueline, Frances Taylor and Erla Larson. *The Whole Way to Allergy Relief & Prevention.* Point Roberts, WA: Hartley & Marks, Inc., 1991.

Levene, G., and Calnan, C. *A Colour Atlas of Dermatology.* London: Wolfe Medical Publications Ltd., 1984.

Lin, Li, and Liu Zhaohui. *Treatment of Psoriasis with Traditional Chinese Medicine.* Hong Kong: Hai Feng Publishing Co., Ltd., 1990.

Mills, Simon, and Kerry Bone. *Principles and Practice of Phytotherapy.* London: Churchill Livingstone, 2000.

Murray, Michael, and Joseph Pizzorno. *Encyclopedia of Natural Medicine, Revised 2nd Edition.* Rocklin, CA: Prima Publishing, 1998.

Murray, Michael. *The Healing Power of Herbs.* Rocklin, CA: Prima Publishing, 1995.

Shen, De-Hui, Xiu-Fen Wu, and Nissi Wang. *Manual of Dermatology in Chinese Medicine.* Seattle, WA: Eastland Press, 1995.

Thomas, Lalitha. *10 Essential Herbs.* Prescott, AZ: Hohm Press, 1992.

Tierney, Lawrence, Stephen McPhee, and Maxine Papadakis, Eds. *Current Medical Diagnosis & Treatment.* Stamford, CT: Appleton & Lange, 1998.

Trowbridge, John, and Morton Walker. *The Yeast Syndrome.* New York, NY: Bantam Books, 1986.

Worwood, Valerie. *The Complete Book of Essential Oils & Aromatherapy.* Novato, CA: New World Library, 1991.

Index

About the Author

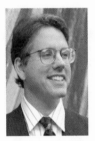

Andrew Gaeddert is one of the foremost herbalists and authorities on complementary and alternative treatments for skin disorders. Mr. Gaeddert has studied nutrition, herbology, and Chinese medicine with masters of herbal medicine from the United States and China. He has been on the protocol team of several scientific studies sponsored by the NIH Office of Alternative Medicine and the University of California. He has lectured at Columbia University, University of San Francisco, Canadian College of Oriental Medicine, and other colleges across the United States. His students have included medical doctors, acupuncturists, herbalists, and other professionals. Mr. Gaeddert is the author of *Healing Digestive Disorders, Digestive Health Now,* and *Chinese Herbs in the Western Clinic,* and the president of Health Concerns. He and his wife live in the San Francisco Bay area.

Books Available
from Get Well Foundation

Healing Skin Disorders

by Andrew Gaeddert   ISBN 1-55643-452-9 $15.95

Filled with self-help stragtegies, treatment protocols, and case studies for all major skin disorders, this book is designed for the professional as well as the layperson. Dietary advice, acupuncture points, herbs, and nutritional supplements make this the most complete book of its kind.

Digestive Health Now

by Andrew Gaeddert   ISBN 1-55643-426-X $12.95

Digestive Health Now explains a four week program that can be completed in the comfort of your own home. There is a meal plan, recipes, and stress relieving techniques. Included are real life success stories of people who have been able to reduce or eliminate medication, and achieve an understanding of what causes symptoms and how to prevent them.

Healing Digestive Disorders

by Andrew Gaeddert   ISBN 1-55643-281-X $15.95

This book by herbalist Andrew Gaeddert lists self-help strategies, treatment protocols, and case studies for all major digestive disorders. Designed for the professional as well as the layperson, *Healing Digestive Disorders* also contains the story of how the author conquered Crohn's disease, a recommended meal plan, workbook section, and acupuncture points.

Chinese Herbs in the Western Clinic

by Andrew Gaeddert   ISBN 0-96382-850-9 $15.95

Chinese Herbs in the Western Clinic recommends formulas by a variety of manufacturers that have been successfully used with thousands of American patients suffering from immune, digestive, gynecological, respiratory disorders, and other commonly seen complaints such as allergies, anxiety, arthritis, back pain, headaches, injury, insomnia and stress. Disorders are alphabetized by Western conditions and indexed by traditional Chinese medical terminology for easy reference while patients are in the office. This book is designed for practitioners.

Sixty Years in Search of Cures

by Dr. Fung Fung and John Fung   ISBN 0-96382-851-7 $15.95

Sixty years in Search of Cures is the autobiography of one of the world's most experienced herbalists, Dr. Fung Fung, who routinely saw 100 to 150 patients per day working in a hospital clinic. This master practitioner with experience in Canton, Hong Kong, Vietnam, and San Francisco, reveals important dietary and lifestyle habits for the general public and herbal prescriptions for the professional herbalist.

Send check or money order payable to Get Well. Include $2.00 per book shipping and handling. California residents add $1.07 sales tax for *Digestive Health Now,* and $1.32 for the other books. Please be sure to write your name and address clearly, and to specify the titles and quantities of each book you want. Allow 4 weeks for delivery.

For trade, bookstore, and wholesale inquiries, contact North Atlantic Books, P.O. Box 12327, Berkeley, CA 94701.

 Get Well Foundation
8001 Capwell Drive, Suite A
Oakland, CA 94621